BIRD FLU

EVERYTHING YOU NEED TO KNOW
ABOUT THE NEXT PANDEMIC

MARC SIEGEL, M.D.

WILEY

John Wiley & Sons, Inc.

To my fearless loving little girl Rebecca

CONTENTS

ACKNOWLEDGMENTS

Bird flu has frightened the world in a hurry, and so this book was written with two major agendas: quality and expediency. I felt the discussion on bird flu required more nuance, more perspective, and to accomplish my goal I had to write this book in a timely manner.

The goal was met because of great sacrifice by my wonderful wife, Luda, who has taken over most of the care of our baby, Samuel, over the past several weeks while I've worked on this project. I hope to make it up to her.

I am appreciative of my patients for their daily discussions with me on bird flu, discussions that inspired much of this book. In some cases, the stories in my office were so striking that they made their way directly onto these pages; in these cases, I have changed patient names to protect their privacy.

I would also like to thank the terrific team at Wiley, who get behind a book for the same reason that I do—because they are passionate about it. I am very grateful for the commitment of the publisher, Kitt Allan, and my editor, Eric Nelson, who have shown great enthusiasm and support. Eric has helped me research and organize this book, and his effort is as important as my own in making sure this book came together. Eric extended himself to every aspect of the project, well beyond an editor's usual role. His assistant, Connie Santisteban, was also crucial to the project. Similarly, my agent, Joelle Delbourgo, has worked many hours coordinating and being supportive. Her wisdom and experience were essential to getting this project off the ground.

My extraordinary friend and practical alter ego, Ken Blaker, has worked tirelessly with me on the manuscript these past few weeks and has contributed countless insights. Ira Berkow, the great sportswriter and columnist for the *New York Times*, has once again offered his wise comments and support.

Mike Onorato, associate director of trade publicity at Wiley, has been generating a lot of excitement for my work. He has helped me greatly in getting my message out there.

John Simko, a consummate production editor with a meticulous eye for detail and a commitment to the English language, pored over this manuscript with an intense effort.

Finally, I would like to thank the media for giving me a forum in which to express myself. Many newspaper and magazine editors and TV and radio producers and hosts have been excited by my perspective and extended themselves to me. The media, while too often generating hysteria, is also often receptive to a greater self-correcting perspective, which is to its credit.

INTRODUCTION

On November 20, 2005, Dr. Anthony Fauci, director of the NIH's National Institutes of Allergy and Infectious Diseases was among a panel of experts interviewed on NBC's *Meet the Press* by moderator Tim Russert.

> Mr. Russert: "Dr. Fauci, how do you explain this to people, that we're here talking about this possibility of a pandemic flu? One, how much of a possibility is it, in your mind? Two, how fearful should people be?"

> Dr. Fauci: "I think it's important to put into context a pandemic flu in general. . . . We had the worst-case scenario in 1918 with . . . 50 million people dead. . . . If you look at the situation in 1968, it was

really dramatically different. It was still a pandemic . . . but relatively speaking, it was rather mild. . . . Sooner or later, the way viruses evolve, we're gonna get another pandemic. It could be a couple years from now; it could be 15 or 20 years from now. If it doesn't happen, that doesn't mean that preparedness went to waste, because sooner or later it's going to happen."

The above quote from Dr. Fauci, one of the world's most prominent infectious disease experts, is compelling, but I worry that most television viewers only really heard one phrase: "50 million people dead." I've written this book because of my concern about the ease with which such potent doses of bird flu jargon can cause public alarms to be sounded. It is too easy to personalize news like this and wrongly believe that you are at immediate risk. Read on, and you will get to see bird flu as the theoretical threat it is in the larger context of disease and public health.

Public health officials need to raise money for their projects. It's easy to justify a specific need by pointing to a greater general threat. For any official who goes this route, though, jumping into the spotlight to draw attention to his or her role to protect us is striking a Faustian bargain. Too often the hype these leaders use to generate public interest leads to the funding going to the wrong places. Preparing for a worst-case scenario is one thing, but devoting most of our attention and money to a rare but potentially devastating short-term outcome doesn't allow us to prepare properly for the long term.

Most of us are greatly motivated by our fear of death. This fear is connected to our fear of the unknown. Most people, when the subject of bird flu comes up, have exactly the same question, worded the same way: "Are we all going to die?" This didn't come out of nowhere. The most prominent statement circulating in the media about bird flu is: "It's not a matter of if, but when." It's a statement made to provide information, but it creates terror and makes us think the grim reaper is looming.

In fact, it is not a given that the current avian influenza virus—the one creating havoc among birds in Asia, killing millions—will mutate sufficiently to pass easily from human to human. It is not a given that even if that necessary mutation occurs, the resulting virus would kill people with the same terrifying speed at which it is killing birds. It is also far from certain, given current technologies and medical care, that even if this bird flu became a bona fide human killer, a mirror image of the 1918 doomsday Spanish flu scenario (or worse) would result.

It is certainly good to be prepared for worst-case scenarios. However, it is naive to think that preparation isn't determined by expectations. If the bird flu mutates this year and begins to take off, then massive emergency government stockpiles would seem to be our best bet. If the far more likely scenario occurs, and the next flu pandemic is still years away, the more prudent direction would be to upgrade our vaccine-making capacity through the use of genetic engineering.

Vaccine manufacturers are afraid of the new technology because it is expensive, and, if hastily applied, there is the risk of lawsuits from potential adverse side effects. Plus, vaccine making is an expensive proposition (with a comparatively low profit margin), especially when you take into account the important need for sterilization. But the current method requires three to six months, which puts us in a poor position to respond after a virus is found to be spreading lethally among humans.

So our public health officials concentrate on the worst-case scenario because they know the safety net is porous. Building up the safety net to the point where it can handle all scenarios requires a significant governmental support of the vaccine industry (i.e., assurances, laws to offset liabilities, billions of dollars) as well as of the emergency response capabilities of our nation's hospitals. In the meantime, our health officials have the difficult task of informing the public in a way that is honest but doesn't provoke public panic.

Unfortunately, fear is its own virus. It spreads more quickly and causes far more damage than does influenza. For example, in the current climate of bird flu fears, if even one chicken in the United States becomes infected with the H5N1 virus, it is likely to cause tremendous damage to the U.S. poultry industry, which provides one third of the world's poultry. Our chickens will be banned, much as European beef has been banned from the United States since the early 1990s because of mad cow disease.

We can learn how not to overreact by looking at recent history. With mad cow disease, for example, the British economy was partly crippled by the overwhelming attention paid to worst-case scenarios and not enough attention paid to the species barrier that protects us from animal infections. Well over one hundred thousand cows had mad cow disease at its peak, but for all the panic it caused, only slightly more than one hundred humans have gotten it by eating beef.

Similarly, SARS choked the Asian economy for fear that it would sweep around the world because we had zero immunity to this emerging virus. It is wise to take precautions, but SARS, like the Ebola and the Marburg viruses, has done a lot more harm from the panic it created than from the actual deaths from the virus. For all the attention it received in 2003, SARS infected approximately seven thousand people worldwide, with zero documented cases in the United States, yet the Asian economy suffered more than $30 billion in lost revenue. Fear was the prevailing virus with SARS, as it threatens to be with bird flu.

Americans are already afraid to eat chicken or turkey, and the Centers for Disease Control and Prevention in Atlanta has received hundreds of calls about whether bird feeders are safe. In the United Kingdom, after a single parrot was found to have the dreaded bird flu virus, chicken consumption was immediately down by a third. In Asia, where chickens walk the streets, bird handling is a more common practice, and there are also ritualistic practices, such as cockfighting, that necessitate close contact (including sharing bird saliva). There have been less than 140 cases so far, with about 70 deaths. Yet despite the low risk, people in Asia are petrified.

In the United States, fear is spreading without any current risk. Many people are afraid to travel to Asia, afraid to eat or touch a bird. This is because we attach ourselves voyeuristically to news reports and because our public health officials—who are trained in laboratory and epidemiological science, not public speaking—have not figured out how to inform us without making us all assume the worst.

The potential economic costs of bird flu are staggering. If the worst case happens and there is a pandemic, there is likely to be economic havoc as normal trade between countries is interrupted. The United States is entirely too dependent on foreign countries for oil, food, and many medications. If a much more likely case occurs and there is no imminent human pandemic, we are still at the mercy of our fears. For example, many millions of dollars will be lost from fear of poultry if even a single chicken comes down with bird flu in the United States. We could become economic outcasts, our trade and tourism stifled.

During a recent typical day in my office when I saw fifteen patients, every single one asked me about bird flu, though several forgot to ask about the diseases I was actually treating them for. Some of the routine questions I received:

"Is there a vaccine?"

"Should I have a ready supply of Tamiflu?"

"Are we all going to die?"

"What do I do if I see a dead bird?"

"What are the typical symptoms of bird flu that I should be on the lookout for?"

All of these questions and many more will be addressed in the course of this book. All of my answers involve putting information into context while learning not to obsess about worst-case scenarios. One of my patients, Mr. Lilly, became so obsessed with bird flu that he stopped eating poultry altogether. Previously he had quit beef for fear of mad cow disease, and fish for fear of mercury. He would remain a vegetarian until he realized that it was almost impossible to find vegetables that weren't genetically engineered.

I was about to tell poor Mr. Lilly that the typical symptoms of bird flu are the same as regular flu, only more severe. But I realized from my work in the media that explaining hypothetical symptoms made them seem more real and imminent and would likely contribute further to his unease.

Instead I tried humor.

"If Chicken Little isn't afraid of the bird flu, why should we be?"

That didn't work. He said that Chicken Little was surely afraid of the bird flu, all birds were, but that the movie had preceded the current concern.

"This virus has been around since the 1950s, and there have been occasional human cases in people with close contact since 1997."

"It's spreading among birds. It's only a matter of when," Lilly said.

There were those public health pronouncements, now in the words of one of my most worried patients.

"Okay," I said. "The symptoms of bird flu are the same as for regular flu only more pronounced. Headache, muscle aches, fever, sore throat, chest congestion. And an irresistible urge to dirty someone's windshield."

He still didn't laugh.

"Very funny," he said. "You're making light of a very serious concern."

That wasn't what I was trying to do. But I was concerned that too much attention to bird flu would take attention away from other essential diseases that were already killing us. In fact, I was invited to an international AIDS conference in early 2006 precisely because its founders were concerned that too much attention to bird flu would take needed resources away from AIDS. Mine was to be the needed voice of reason to explain that avian influenza is a great concern because of what it *could do*, whereas AIDS (more than 3 million deaths worldwide yearly), tuberculosis (2 million deaths yearly), and malaria (1 million deaths yearly), are concerns because of what they already *are doing*.

And in my office practice in New York City, there are many less mysterious diseases than the wanton bird flu virus that are already killing my patients. (It might be a good idea to avoid fried chicken, but because it's fried—not because it's chicken.) The mundane killers—obesity, heart disease, cancer, stroke—combine to kill well over 3 million in the United States every year. People worrying about bird flu add stress to the equation and are thereby more at risk for these ordinary diseases. And people who worry are more likely to get into car accidents, which kill over a million people every year around the world.

Ironically, AIDS, which may lose needed attention in favor of the hot "bug du jour" that is bird flu, is itself used as one of the justifications for the intense public obsession with bird flu. "We let the horses out of the barn with AIDS; it was halfway around the world before anyone in the scientific community took it seriously. We're not going to let this happen again"—or so the argument on behalf of the full-court press goes.

On the other side of the argument is the realization that the AIDS rationale has been used previously to justify public health reactions to killer bees, mad cow disease, anthrax, West Nile virus, and SARS, reactions out of proportion to the risk at the time. Public health predictions have had a low batting average. Previous failings to predict AIDS in time are hardly justifications for over-reacting to everything else, in part because resources are still needed for AIDS, a massive worldwide killer.

People in government also make the claim that since Hurricane Katrina caused such devastation and we were so unprepared for it, we therefore have to prepare for

8

bird flu now, before it is too late. But Katrina doesn't justify sounding all the warning bells for everything. Katrina was a likely scenario, not a worst case. Those levees in New Orleans were likely to break in response to a hurricane with the force of Katrina. In fact, it was partly because the Federal Emergency Management Agency (FEMA) had been placed under the wing of the Department of Homeland Security that we were more ready for bioterror than for a naturally occurring disaster that was more or less inevitable.

Preparedness means taking into account both the likelihood of an event's occurring as well as the number of people who would be affected by it. Preparedness means considering the worst-case scenario while mostly preparing for the more likely ones. Communication of risk to the public includes learning the language of probabilities, so the public learns how to tell the difference between an unlikely event and a likely one.

The major difficulty with achieving perspective about bird flu and the associated risk is due to the fact that scientists who have spent their lives working in laboratories are ill equipped to transmit their ideas at press conferences. In the era of twenty-four-hour cable news, messages are instantly transmitted all over the world, and the impact is enormous. Intensity about a virus, productive when confronting a microscope, is too likely to be misinterpreted over the airwaves as signifying that danger is imminent.

Most people, when they think of bird flu, have a different movie in mind than *Chicken Little*. Somehow, birds scare us. They swoop and have beady little eyes, long talons, and beaks, and we never know where they are going to be at any given moment. Alfred Hitchcock understood that, and he used the narrative of dangerous birds taking over a whole town quite effectively in *The Birds*.

But Hitchcock also noted that the reason he was comfortable scaring people for entertainment was that at the end of the show the projector was turned off and everyone got to go back home, back to safe, mundane, regular life.

Unfortunately, with the bird flu scare there is no going home. Diseases that scare us out of proportion to their ability to infect us (except for the worst-case scenario) stay in our thoughts, and we believe that they are going to happen to us. Fear is not rational, but it is very powerful. Once it is turned on, it is very difficult to turn it off.

Part I

FACTS
AND
FICTIONS

1

BIRD FLU BASICS

What is bird flu?

All bird flus are influenza A. Influenza A is primarily a respiratory virus, causing coughing, congestion, sore throat, muscle aches, fatigue, and fever in most species it infects.

This strain (also called the H5N1 virus) surfaced in Hong Kong eight years ago, although it may have been around for four decades previous to this. It has mostly been affecting Asian poultry. When tested in the laboratory, it has been found to be quite deadly, killing ten out of ten chick embryos against which it was tested. It is difficult to tell how many birds it has killed in Asia, though, because millions of birds have been killed by humans to prevent its spread. As soon as one chicken develops symptoms, it is killed along with all the chickens that may have come in contact with it.

It appears to be quite deadly to humans as well, although in Hong Kong in 1997 many humans reportedly developed antibodies to the virus and did not get sick. There is concern that if the virus mutated, it could cause a pandemic because we do not have built-up immunity to it. This mutation could occur either at random or if the virus mixes its DNA with a human flu virus inside a pig or a human. But it's also quite possible (in fact it's even more likely) that it may never mutate at all or that if it does mutate, the mutated virus would result in a much less severe illness in humans.

What is influenza?

Influenza is a virus. Unlike bacteria, which are single cells, a virus is not a full cell and cannot reproduce on its own. To reproduce, a virus infects a cell and uses the resources of that cell. Essentially, a virus is just a sack of genetic material enclosed by a protein envelope. Viruses don't even fit the definition of "alive," though most scientists agree that they are.

There are two types of viruses: DNA (deoxyribonucleic acid) and RNA (ribonucleic acid). Influenza is an RNA virus. Influenza comes in two main varieties: A and B. (It also comes in a C, which rarely causes illness.) Influenza A viruses are found in many different animals, including ducks, chickens, pigs, whales, horses, and seals. Influenza B viruses circulate widely only among humans and generally do not make us as sick as influenza A does.

Influenza A viruses are divided into subtypes based on two bumpy proteins on the surface of the virus: the hemagglutinin (H) and the neuraminidase (N). These two identifying proteins are why the current bird flu is referred to as H5N1. There are 16 different hemagglutinin subtypes and 9 different neuraminidase subtypes, all of which have been found among influenza A viruses in wild birds. H5 and H7 subtypes include all the current pathogenic strains.

How does influenza spread and what complications does it cause?

Influenza is spread by airborne droplets and is inhaled into the respiratory tract. It incubates in the body from one to four days before a person feels ill. Complications tend to occur in the very young, in the elderly, and in patients with chronic cardiopulmonary diseases. The major complication of flu is pneumonia from influenza itself, or bacterial pneumonia from pneumococcus or haemophilus.

How is influenza diagnosed?

Influenza is most commonly diagnosed by recognizing symptoms or by direct examination of respiratory secretions. Blood examination (serology) can determine exposure.

What is a pandemic?

A pandemic occurs when many people in several different regions of the world are suffering from a specific illness at the same time. Human pandemics may occur when we are exposed to a virus strain for the first time and we lack immunity to it.

Is there a bird flu test?

The current bird flu is diagnosed by testing the blood for antibodies to the H5N1 strain. The test is 100 percent accurate, though it doesn't tell how sick a bird (or a person) is. Transmission from bird to human is possible but rare, and almost exclusively from close or frequent contact.

How does a bird get it?

It's endemic in birds, especially waterfowl like geese and ducks. It's usually a benign infection of the gastrointestinal or respiratory tracts of waterfowl, and it has existed in birds for many thousands of years. It can pass from wild birds to the poultry on farms when they come into contact, and certain strains, known as pathogenic avian influenza, make these domestic birds very sick. The flu virus mutates frequently, changing its genetics, but it rarely goes through the changes that allow it to routinely infect mammals.

How do birds transmit it to each other?

Birds transmit viruses the same way we do: by sneezing, coughing, and touching other birds.

Is there a cure once you have it?

There is no cure for any influenza for either birds or people. The body's own immune system fights it, and antiviral drugs such as amantadine, ramitidine, Relenza, and Tamiflu are probably all effective against H5N1 bird flu, though the degree of effectiveness hasn't been shown. Although there have been over a hundred reported human cases in Asia, it's not clear if more people have it, but it just didn't make them sick.

With most cases of the annual flu virus, the vast majority of people get better without serious treatment as their immune system fights off the virus. It's the cases where prolonged recuperation or hospitalization becomes necessary that worry doctors.

How fast would a human pandemic spread?

There is concern that air travel would accelerate transmission around the world, although scientific recognition of the mutation early on and the worldwide communication network could help to slow its spread by warning people.

What should I be doing to protect myself?

People are concerned about the possibility of a coming pandemic. The way this information has been communicated in the media and via several of our public health officials carries the message that something major is in the offing. This makes a worst case seem like the only case.

In fact, the government has a reason to consider worst-case scenarios as it attempts to protect us, but we need to consider that a massive pandemic may well *not* be in the offing. As I suggest here specific measures of personal preparation, I, too, must be careful about hidden messages. When I advise a certain kind of preparation, I must consider if I am inadvertently suggesting that something must be about to happen.

I do not think a massive bird flu pandemic that kills many millions of people worldwide is about to happen, for reasons that I will go into throughout this book. The major reason is that, as with mad cow disease, which has killed hundreds of thousands of cows but only a little over a hundred people, we are currently protected by a species barrier. For bird flu to pass human to human, further changes in its structure have to occur. Influenza viruses change frequently, but this form of H5N1 appears to have been around since the 1950s, and in the eight years that it has infected millions of birds (1997–2005), documented human cases have been rare (less than 150 clinical infections with 70 deaths at the time of this writing). We don't know how many thousands have developed antibodies to this virus and not gotten sick from it, so it may not be as deadly as it seems to be to humans. If it mutates sufficiently to infect us routinely, it may do so in a way that causes it to be far less lethal.

Should I prepare emergency supplies of food and water just in case?

Absolutely not. We've been asking one another this question ever since experts told us that the year 2000 bug in our computers would shut down communications and banking nationwide.

Sinister things scare us out of proportion to their actual risk of affecting us, and we respond, quite naturally, by wanting to be afraid. But bird flu can be seen as one in a long line of things we've been warned about, and for which we supposedly need some kind of "safe room" with an ample supply of food and water just in case.

In one sense, there is little difference between a grizzled

terrorist and a mysterious bird flu. Both scare us beyond their reach, beyond the likelihood that they will hurt us. In the wake of 9/11, our leaders have been playing Chicken Little. First it was anthrax, then West Nile virus, then smallpox, then SARS. In each case we were warned that we had no immunity and could be at great risk. In each case there was no accountability going forward, no "We're sorry, we got this one wrong, but we just wanted to prepare you just in case."

It is difficult to trust an official who scared us unnecessarily about smallpox to inform us contextually about bird flu, even if that person is a devoted scientist.

The national psyche has been damaged by all these false alarms. We each make risk assessments, scanning our environment for potential threats, worrying more and more of the time. The emotional center of the brain, the amygdala, cannot process fear and courage at the exact same moment. If we could train ourselves to filter out dangers that don't threaten us by setting our default drives to courage or caring or laughter, we'd be a lot better off.

We don't need emergency supplies of food, we need leaders and information sources we can trust. In a true emergency, our satellite-driven communication system will be our ally, as long as the warnings we receive are accurate and not overblown. Fear is our ultimate warning system, designed to protect us against imminent danger. Our fear responses should not be overdetermined.

By jumping from one fear to the next, we create a climate of distrust. One of my patients told me that he is readying for the coming flu pandemic not only by stockpiling food but by keeping two rifles, ammunition, and a trained German Shepherd at the ready. He envisions a scenario where he may have to barricade himself into his house in order to protect his wife and his two young children. He expects people to be dropping dead in the streets of flu, and he anticipates strangers trying to get into his house to hide from the virus.

This Hitchcockian image is not only extremely unlikely, it contributes to a pattern of thinking that pits us against one another. It is only a half stop from this kind of irrational fright to deep-rooted prejudices where everyone is "the other" and the only way to maintain safety is to cordon off your house.

Should I wash my hands more frequently?

Hand washing is always a good idea as a protection against all respiratory and gastrointestinal viruses, from the common cold to influenza to mononucleosis. Good sanitary practices are essential to not getting the flu if you are in very close contact with it, but more than that, good hygiene is important in not getting any kind of virus or bacteria.

In the fall of 2005, the purchase of hand sanitizers was up almost tenfold. I'm sure this is a response to the fear of getting bird flu. Bird flu is not here, and frequent hand washing or use of sanitizers is a way to reassure yourself in the short term that you are doing something to protect yourself. I would never discourage hand cleansing, but keep in mind that any quick remedy for bird flu fears also reinforces the notion that bird flu is almost here, when there is no evidence to support this. The same is true for avoiding poultry. It may make some people feel safer for a brief moment, but it also reinforces the misconception that our poultry supply is at risk, when it isn't.

Are there specific medical supplies I should stockpile against bird flu? What about Tamiflu?

There is currently no need to personally stockpile anti-virals like Tamiflu (Roche pharmaceuticals) for protection against bird flu. Tamiflu has been tested against this bird flu in mice and is probably effective in humans as well at reducing symptoms, but the doses would probably have to be higher for bird flu than for the usual flu to be effective. It is generally effective when taken in the first forty-eight hours after symptoms begin. A recent study suggests that Tamiflu stockpiles for 25 percent of the population would be sufficient to protect us during a colossal pandemic.

Currently there is no indication for taking Tamiflu for anyone other than perhaps a bird handler or cockfighting organizer in areas of Asia where bird flu is endemic. As with Cipro for anthrax, there is the tendency for fear to create a dependency need for a pill that is not particularly necessary. Not only that, but personal stockpiles remove the physician as an essential filter to decide when a med should be taken. Tamiflu is a well-tolerated drug with nausea as its most common side effect, but taking it when there isn't a situation of true risk from exposure or an ongoing flu is a wasteful use of the drug. Amantadine, an older antiviral drug that is also effective against many strains of influenza A, has been shown in a recent study to have developed a 12 percent resistance to flu viruses because of overuse.

Tamiflu is an expensive drug that has approximately a three-year shelf life, and since bird flu most likely won't mutate to a form that can routinely infect humans over the next few years, the chances are that if you stockpile

Tamiflu, you will either misuse it or be compelled to throw it away when it is out of date.

Plus, even if you stockpiled it, without a physician's instructions you'd never know when the appropriate time to take it would be. When there's a rumor of a sick parrot in a cage at LaGuardia? When a human gets it in Madagascar? The first time someone sneezes in your vicinity near the poultry counter of your local super-market?

How can I protect myself in general against airborne viruses?

This is an important question, and the same basic precautions against all respiratory viruses are applicable to human flu as well as to bird flu if it were to mutate to a human-to-human form. First, frequent hand washing decreases the spread of flu viruses. Be conscious of how often you shake hands or casually kiss someone at a party. These friendly practices spread viruses such as the flu. A sneeze or a cough can propel a virus ten to twelve feet. Cigarette smoke also spreads respiratory viruses, so smokers (and smokers' friends) have to be very careful when they are sick to not blow smoke into a crowded room.

Isolating sick people is the best protection against the spread of flu. Unfortunately, a patient may be spreading the virus for several days before becoming clinically ill. Close contacts of people who are ill should anticipate the possibility of getting sick and in the "window period" should take extra precautions in terms of limiting personal contacts.

What about the yearly flu vaccine?

The yearly flu vaccine is helpful in terms of introducing a "herd immunity," which may protect high-risk groups (the elderly, asthmatics, those with emphysema and diabetes, infants, pregnant women, and the immunocompromised) by decreasing the amount of circulating flu virus. But a British study this year showed only a mild effect on saving elderly lives.

This result is consistent with a previous National Institutes of Health (NIH) review of the elderly's response to the flu vaccine over the past three decades. But the vaccine is still recommended for those over sixty-five, as it appears to decrease the risk of getting severe complications of the flu, such as pneumonia, which can lead to hospitalization. I recommend the yearly flu shot to anyone in a high-risk group, and I suggest it as an option for anyone who is over fifty or has any chronic illness.

Unfortunately, because the flu vaccine is still made by cultivating the virus in chicken-egg culture (fifty-year-old technology), those with egg allergies often cannot tolerate it.

And as far as anyone knows, the yearly flu vaccine does not offer protection against bird flu. This is subject to some debate, because there is crossover protection from one strain of influenza to another, but significant protection against the H5N1 strain has not been shown. As I will discuss later in this book, there is ongoing research into the development of a single flu vaccine that will cover all strains, including H5N1, and will offer protection for at least ten years. If such a vaccine were commercially available, it would certainly alter prevention strategies for pandemics.

In the meantime, the current flu vaccine is good for only one year. It is made this way in part because the predominant yearly flu strain changes from one year to the next. Epidemiologists track it in South America and Asia at least six months before it comes to the United States. Scientists try to make a vaccine that they feel will best match the predominant yearly strain.

Patients in any of the high-risk categories should also be considered for pneumovax. The pneumonia vaccine lasts for five to ten years and covers twenty-three different strains of pneumococcal pneumonia, a common and potentially life-threatening complication of the flu. Approximately 50 percent of the deaths during a flu season are from pneumonia, the vast majority of which are from the bacteria pneumococcus, which is generally covered by the pneumonia vaccine.

If there is a bird flu pandemic, the pneumonia vaccine will be a useful adjunct, in that it will protect people from a serious secondary complication that leads to about half of the deaths.

In the meantime, an op-ed in the *New York Times* on November 30, 2005, had my phone ringing with urgent calls for pneumovax. Though some of my patients were embarrassed to admit it, the article—though it had been attempting to show the value of protection against pneumonia as part of a prevention strategy against flu—had also inadvertently sent an implicit message that a pandemic was in the offing. This converted the pneumonia vaccine to yet another prop or treatment of the fear of bird flu, rather than of bird flu itself.

Should I take a bird flu vaccine?

Currently, there is no commercially available bird flu vaccine for human use. One has been developed for the H5N1 virus, and the NIH is currently testing it in an elderly population of volunteers with good results so far. But since the current H5N1 bird flu hasn't mutated to a form that can routinely affect people, there is currently no indication for this vaccine.

If H5N1 does mutate, it may change to a form that is only partly affected by the current vaccine. In H5N1's current form, it appears that high doses (given in two separate shots) are necessary to achieve immunity.

A similar vaccine has been developed that is quite effective in birds. Over 20 million birds have been vaccinated in China to date in an attempt to help control H5N1 while it is still primarily in the bird population.

What are the chances of bird flu getting me?

Right now, the chances are almost nonexistent for anyone who does not have intimate contact with birds in Asia. And even for Asian bird handlers, the chances are very slim. The concern about the disease itself is based on the fact that the H5N1 pathogenic avian influenza is a very aggressive killer of birds, and as it spreads in birds, it increases the worldwide viral load of this particular virus.

Because flus change rapidly, it is feared that the more virus there is, the greater the chance it will mutate spontaneously or acquire the necessary genetic material from exchange with another flu virus inside a pig or a human.

But the chances of this occurring are very small for any given period of time and are not directly proportional to the number of infected birds.

In the meantime, it is important to realize that not a single bird in the United States has been found to have this pathogenic avian influenza. As of this writing, no migratory birds have yet brought it to Alaska, and even if that dreaded event were to happen, most of America's poultry is not killed in the open where H5N1 can easily spread. And even in Asia, where birds freely walk the streets of many villages and towns and outbreaks in birds continue to occur (twenty-four outbreaks in China this year alone, and in May H5N1 killed 10 percent of the world's bar-headed geese), eating cooked poultry is safe. Casual contact with birds will not give you the flu. You are protected by a species barrier; it is very difficult for you to get this virus from birds, even in parts of Asia where the virus is endemic in birds.

Bird feeders are safe; pigeons are safe; and if you encounter a dead bird, do not assume that it died of bird flu. If you are worried to that extent, it is a sign that fear is becoming virulent, rather than that H5N1 is spreading.

I am so bombarded with bird flu warnings in the media that I feel I should do something. What should I do?

Eat right and get plenty of exercise—the same things your doctor always tells you. Right now, the best thing you can do is to not obsess about it and to continue with your regular routines. I hope that this book will provide a perspective on bird flu that will counter excess emotion with reason. Avian influenza has been around for thousands of years, and thousands of varieties of the virus exist, a few of which mutate sufficiently to affect humans. Many pathogenic strains never make that jump. Rarely a pandemic strain develops, the last two of which (in 1957 and 1968) have only been slightly worse than the yearly flu season in the United States.

It behooves the world's scientists, animal experts, and public health officials alike to do their best to try to control H5N1 in birds. That job hasn't worked nearly well enough to this point. Improved international cooperation is crucial. Better funding for bird culling and vaccination programs is crucial. But currently, the problem is far more a bird problem than it is a human problem.

If a fire occurred away from your house, your best protection would be to put out the fire rather than to immediately build a firewall around your house.

Currently, fear of bird flu is much more a human problem than bird flu itself. Fear is intended to be a warning system to protect us against imminent dangers. It is good that we know about bird flu, that we are learning as a society that it has a potential to expand into a problem that can threaten us, but in the meantime, while it remains remote and theoretical, excess worry or turning on our fear radar unnecessarily can do us more harm than good.

It is wise for people to be interested in their health, not waiting until illness strikes to show concern. But personal attention is better paid to a healthy lifestyle and a display of positive emotions like courage and caring than to worry about health threats that may never materialize.

Right now, there is no physical protection necessary for humans against bird flu, either here in the United

States, where the H5N1 disease doesn't exist even in birds, or even in Asia, where cooking poultry kills flu viruses and casual contact with birds is safe.

Is travel to Asia safe?

If you're not planning on staying on a chicken farm and interacting intimately with the chickens, you're good to go.

There have been twenty-four outbreaks of bird flu in China this year and several more in Indonesia. Twenty million birds have been vaccinated against bird flu, and many millions more have been culled. The UN Food and Agriculture Organization (FAO) is engaged in a multi-country program designed to increase awareness throughout Asia. To date, bird flu has claimed forty-two human lives in Vietnam, thirteen in Thailand, nine in Indonesia, four in Cambodia, and two in China. The virus remains extremely difficult for humans to catch.

"The FAO believes that eliminating avian influenza among poultry can delay H5N1 virus turning into a form that would create a human pandemic," Serge Verniau, an FAO representative in Afghanistan, said at a recent workshop there. The FAO has begun working closely with the World Health Organization and the World Bank to promote a regional network for improving surveillance and diagnosis of the disease in both birds and the rare human. It also hopes to encourage the exchange of information on the occurrence of the disease and on the lessons learned.

In the meantime, travel to Asia remains quite safe. The occasional human case has been the result of close contact between birds and people in primitive agrarian settings. But for tourists traveling to the major cities and towns, there is no risk of acquiring bird flu whatsoever.

Even for people who live in the small villages where the outbreaks have occurred, the risks are remote beyond the food handlers and the bird handlers. As for the birds, even though much Asian poultry is free ranging and may come in contact with other birds, potentially spreading the infection prior to being killed for food (the incubation period in birds is seven to ten days), according to Dr. Ron De Haven of the U.S. Department of Agriculture (USDA), there is a growing surveillance network that is serologically testing thousands of birds in the area of an outbreak.

Cooking poultry kills the H5N1 virus 100 percent of the time, so eating cooked poultry in Asia is completely safe.

What are the chances of bird flu coming to the United States?

It is possible in birds, and very unlikely in humans.

The USDA is working with the FAO and the Organization of International Epizootics to promote biosecurity throughout the world. It is very unlikely that a live bird will pass bird flu (H5N1) to North America, though bird smugglers do exist. According to Dr. De Haven, it is far more likely that some chilled or frozen poultry, mislabeled or smuggled from Asia, will be brought here containing H5N1. This is very difficult to control and is also of minimal risk, beyond the panic it might cause. If a piece of dead infected poultry was brought here, the virus would be destroyed as soon as it was cooked and would not be transmitted to humans or other animals.

The chances of an infected human bringing bird flu to the United States on a plane is practically nonexistent, simply because there are so few cases of human bird flu. But there may be many more subclinical cases than are known, since routine serological testing of contacts of the few human cases has not been routinely done. But even if someone brought bird flu here on a plane, it would not spread, because there is no human-to-human transmission with bird flu in its current state.

A third possible way that bird flu could arrive here, perhaps the most likely, is through Alaska. Unlike the Middle East, there are no regular migratory bird pathways from Asia to the United States. But Pacific flyaway birds can occasionally make it across Siberia to Alaska. Since waterfowl (ducks and geese) are reservoirs for avian influenzas, and many species of ducks in particular can be asymptomatic carriers, it is conceivable that H5N1 could show up in Alaska and from there make its way down the West Coast or across Canada.

However, there is much less contact between migratory birds and poultry in the United States than in Asia. Most of our poultry here is commercially raised, kept and killed inside buildings, with little or no access to wild circulating flocks. The chance of bird flu circulating among our poultry is therefore much less than in Asia.

What if the worst-case scenario does occur and the H5N1 bird flu does mutate to a form that can infect me? What if it comes here to the United States in that altered form? What would I do then?

In the first place, as I hope to establish further in this book, worrying about the worst-case scenario all the time is bad for our health and takes our attention away from more pressing health concerns that we really can do something about. Secondly, there is little any of us can do right now to protect ourselves from an unmutated bird flu that doesn't directly threaten us.

But if this bird flu does mutate and explode into the next 1918-style pandemic, there will be plenty of worthwhile precautions we can take.

First, we can stay calm and listen to public health advisories over the airwaves. It will be important that a consistent, accurate, noninflammatory message be delivered by the CDC and by state and local health agencies. Today's worldwide communication network, including satellite and Internet, can be an enormous asset in keeping people informed and advised at the time of a great infectious-disease catastrophe.

Second, it would be important to reduce crowds as much as possible. One of the greatest reasons for the rapid spread of the Spanish flu was the public meetings and crowds and rallies throughout World War I that facilitated the spread of the H1N1 virus.

If a massive pandemic spread today, we would be advised to not meet in public, to isolate sick patients, to obey travel advisories, and above all, to not panic.

Panic leads to the greatest amount of viral spread, because when people panic, they tend to take fewer precautions. Washing hands frequently, not coughing or sneezing on people, and not shaking hands or sharing drinking cups or silverware are all crucial methods to control viral spread.

In 1918 people didn't understand what viruses were or how best to contain them. Many people—especially the poor—lived crowded, unsanitary lives.

We also have medical treatments today that will be crucial in preventing deaths in a large pandemic. Patients with heart disease, asthma, diabetes, emphysema, and AIDS would all be much more at risk of dying if they lost access to their regular medical treatment.

Treatments for these underlying conditions that were lacking in 1918 and that led to the greatest loss of life will be lifesaving now. Pneumonia will need to be recognized right away and treated aggressively with antibiotics. Since pneumonia and other bacterial infections such as sinusitis were listed on the death certificates of over half of those who died of the Spanish flu, it is likely that early intervention with antibiotics (which hadn't been discovered in 1918) will reduce the death rates dramatically in any flu pandemic that happens now.

Maintaining national and regional supplies of medications will be paramount, especially as regular trade and business will likely be hampered by the pandemic and the need for strict travel guidelines.

Was the 1918 virus a bird flu?

Yes, it was, and research over the past decade has revealed that it made the jump directly from birds to humans via mutation. However, and this is something to always keep in mind, it was not a big killer of birds before this mutation occurred. There's not necessarily any connection between what's deadly in birds and what's deadly in humans.

Why are some projections for this bird flu worse than that of 1918?

As long as we're talking about worst-case scenarios, you should know that public health officials are concerned about the possibility of a worse pandemic at some point for the following reasons: (1) The world is much more densely populated now than in 1918, with more of this population concentrated in the cities. Denser population is more conducive to the spread of a respiratory virus like influenza. (2) There are more elderly, chronically ill, and immuno-compromised individuals now than in 1918. These groups are more at risk of dying of the flu, although, as I will discuss in a later chapter, it was the young who died in the highest numbers in 1918 of the Spanish flu. (3) Plane travel increases the ease of viral spread from one corner of the globe to another, contributing to a pandemic. (4) The virus itself is currently far more deadly than the 1918 strain, which killed about 2.5 percent of the people it infected. (Of course, the lethality of the virus should diminish significantly if the virus mutates. In order to mutate to a form that can infect us, it must sacrifice some of its ability to kill.)

It's also important to understand that there are many people out there who mean well when they give these projections. A scientist looking for funding on how to significantly improve our vaccine capabilities may only be trying to scare people into understanding why long-term planning is important. Ironically, panicked politicians are likely to run right past him, funding short-term solutions that treat a created societal inflammation.

How should the government prepare to protect us against the worst case as well as against more likely scenarios?

The first thrust should be made toward trying to control bird flu in the bird population. Most people who hear about bird flu vastly overestimate how bad this is likely to be for humans, while underestimating how terrible it already is for birds. This particular pathogenic, H5N1, has been spreading and reappearing in birds in Southeast Asia since 1997, and it is quite deadly in birds. Recently it has spread to Turkey and China, and all attempts to stamp it out completely have failed.

No one knows what the risk is of it mutating to a form that can routinely be transmitted among humans, but Dr. De Haven, the USDA's chief administrator of the Animal and Plant Health Inspection Service, and many other animal and public health experts believe that the best strategy is to decrease the worldwide viral load by vaccinating large populations of birds in countries where the disease has appeared and culling birds in affected populations. The USDA has allotted over $4 million for a bird biosecurity outreach program in Asia to keep infected birds from coming to the United States, but far more money is needed. Billions are proposed to be spent on human preparation, but if more were spent on controlling a bird disease in birds, humans might never need the protection.

Dr. De Haven has been meeting regularly with the FAO, the Organization of International Epizootics, and leaders from the World Bank, who are now to begin to provide funding.

On the human side of the equation, it is wise for our government and governments around the world to work together. Our CDC is combining with the WHO to build a worldwide network that tracks emerging diseases and recognizes and prepares for potential pandemics. If bird flu is the disease that fuels that response and improves that network, that is a good thing.

At the same time, resources should not be taken away from the current worldwide killers (malnutrition, AIDS, tuberculosis, malaria, heart disease, schistosomiasis, hepatitis) to provide excess resources only for bird flu worst-case scenarios.

The current H5N1 bird flu should be targeted mainly in birds, because the risk to humans is currently very slight. And nothing would reduce the risk of its killing people directly or mutating into a deadly human virus like cutting back on the pool of birds that have it. Preparation for human pandemics can be of a more general nature, because we don't know what pathogen will cause the next major pandemic or even whether it will be a bird flu.

Here are some major priorities for governmental protection and preparation that I will describe throughout this book:

- Improve the hospital infrastructure and include emergency response plans for influenza as well as for other pathogens.

- Upgrade vaccine manufacture using twenty-first-century genetic technology, cell culture, and DNA splicing, with the goal to improve response time. If 100 million doses of a vaccine for a specific flu could be manufactured in a month or two, as is possible with the latest techniques, then the need for government stockpiling for a particular bird flu such as H5N1 would be much less.

- While developing these new vaccine strategies, put together emergency stockpiles against certain pathogens, such as H5N1, where the effects of a human pandemic would be greatest.

- Discourage personal stockpiles. Personal stockpiles will lead to improper use of a drug like Tamiflu, when no current need exists. Patients won't know when it is right to take this drug without a doctor's advice.

- Public health officials must learn a new language for communicating risk. It is crucial to learn how to correctly convey to the public that a threat over a given period of time is very small but worth taking seriously because the worst case is devastating. Proper preparation can be accomplished without panicking the public. It should not be necessary to alarm the public as a ploy to get funding for disaster planning. This strategy frequently backfires, as money gets wasted on only the worst case and there is little left for the more likely threats. Since we can't worry or prepare for everything, we should expend our national resources rationally.

- Revamp the Federal Emergency Management Agency (FEMA). This agency has become so dysfunctional because its focus has become bioterror, which is far more likely to affect a smaller number of people than an influenza outbreak would. FEMA would function better if it were back on its own, separate from Homeland Security, preparing strategies for all major disasters, not just worst-case scenarios.

  An example of how far FEMA has fallen is its own Web site, which uses a hermit crab as its educational mascot for children. It shows the shell being burned up or blown off and the crab crawling away to safety no matter what the disaster. But a hermit crab is hardly an inspiring creature for our children, even if it does survive. Whatever happened to our bald eagle? Is FEMA somehow afraid it will invoke images of bird flu?

- In the United States, we are dependent on other societies for many of our major products. In the event of a major pandemic, we might be cut off, so our government needs to work on improving its domestic supply of essential goods, from food to energy to medicines. Fear and panic are bound to accelerate this need of domestic production in a large pandemic, because in a climate of fear an afflicted country is likely to be shunned by the rest of the world. (SARS is an example of this, and its numbers were quite small compared to a major flu pandemic). Dr. David Fedson, the former medical director of Aventis-Pasteur, said recently at a bird flu conference held by the Council on Foreign Relations in November 2005, "Do we realize that most of the diagnostic kits we have for flu in this country right now have component parts that come from outside the country or the entire kit is assembled outside the country? Supply chains are very thin. We'll lose our ability to diagnose this [flu] overnight when the pandemic begins because there is no surge capacity, no inventory capacity for making diagnostic kits."

What are the essentials of President Bush's plan for bird flu pandemic preparedness?

The plan calls for a $7.1 billion total expenditure. The president proposes that $2 billion of this would be devoted to stockpiling antiviral medications and 20 million doses of an experimental vaccine against the bird flu strain H5N1. $2.7 billion would go toward vaccine research and upgrading our methods of vaccine manufacture. Federal dollars would be invested in an international flu-surveillance network, and federal funding to state and local public health agencies would be boosted by $100 million.

Critics of the plan say that far too little is designated for the state and local agencies or for fighting bird flu in Asia, where it is currently (only $251 million would be spent overseas). Critics also have complained that the plan doesn't provide for improving the hospital infrastructure for disaster response. According to Dr. Irwin Redlener, associate dean and director of the National Center for Disaster Preparedness at the Mailman School of Public Health at Columbia University (speaking from the audience at the avian influenza conference held by the Council on Foreign Relations in November 2005), "7.1 billion focused mostly on antivirals and vaccine development, which is fine, but less than seven percent of that budget could be construed as going towards anything that would help bolster a very ailing hospital system in the United States. Which in fact would be the only recourse that we would have if, in fact, we're dealing with a race against time, which we are. And if it becomes real that we get a pandemic prior to the development of sufficient capacity to contain, to vaccinate and to treat with specific antivirals, then all we have left is a health and hospital system . . . we'll find that we don't have sufficient isolation beds, intensive care beds, ventilators, et cetera, et cetera."

Watching cable news, I have the impression that something is about to happen. But many experts talk about long-term preparedness. How is that going to help me now?

Dr. Michael Osterholm, director of the Center for Infectious Disease Research and Policy at the University of Minnesota, answered this question when speaking at the Council on Foreign Relations bird flu conference in November 2005: "Much of the preparation that we need to do for pandemic influenza is long-term preparedness; it's not overnight, immediate-reaction preparedness. . . . I think what's happened in the last six weeks has been a media on steroids, that basically went from no attention to this, or very limited attention. But then all of a sudden everybody discovered it after Katrina and the intersection between lack-of-preparedness and now-we-need-another-story created this. And what we need to do is even that out; we need to get perspective. . . . And hopefully we can get back to a point where we will see that this is really necessary preparedness."

2

THE HISTORY OF
BIRD FLU

Influenza pandemics in perspective

In 1997, an apparent new strain of influenza A broke out
in Hong Kong in birds (it was discovered later that this
strain may have dated back to the 1950s). At the time,
local officials thought they were able to get it under control. But when it reappeared a few years later, this strain
(H5N1), perhaps because it was continuing to mutate,
spread more quickly and over a larger geographical area
than most previous influenzas, decimating the feathered
population in its wake. Millions of birds were killed.
Scientists became worried about their inability to prepare
for and manage, let alone eliminate, this threat.

For chickens, this was easily the most terrifying thing
to happen since Colonel Sanders opened for business. For
humans, the risk has remained mostly theoretical.

The H5N1 virus has remained primarily an avian virus, and the population it has decimated is primarily poultry. At least seventy people have died, which is inarguably tragic, but the total number is very small compared to the toll of almost every other disease currently taking human lives.

But you can also see why, if the virus were ever to affect humans in the same way it has birds, it could be calamitous. Everyone who follows this story needs to understand both sides of the discussion. The fear surrounding avian flu comes not from what's currently happening, but from what-if scenarios.

People worry: What if the disease becomes a human virus that spreads just as quickly and remains deadly? It's an important question, but for nonscientists it's easy to become confused about how likely the pandemic scenario is. We need to be in awe of the potential for damage, while learning to understand why the likelihood of the worst case coming to pass is awfully low.

Images of the Spanish flu terrify us. Though times have certainly changed, and we are protected to a large extent by modern medicine, it is still reasonable to be awed and humbled by the effects of the Spanish flu and to wonder whether another bird flu could one day be as bad for humans or even worse. The Spanish flu was the most deadly disease outbreak in recorded history.

The Spanish flu

By 1918, most of the nations of Europe, along with the United States and much of the Middle East, were at war. The United States had entered World War I, or the Great War, on the side of the Allied powers—France,

Great Britain, Italy, Japan, and Russia. They were engaged in a broad and bloody trench war with the Central powers—Germany, Austria-Hungary, and Turkey.

The old empires were crumbling, the older order was destabilized, and despite a strong vein of isolationism among the American people, President Woodrow Wilson had declared war on Germany.

In early March 1918, before a significant number of American GIs had even arrived in the killing fields of Europe, a few soldiers at Camp Funston, Kansas, came down with the flu. Within days hundreds of soldiers at the camp were sick. At the time, and for many years afterward, no one knew where this new strain of the influenza virus had come from, and the medical personnel at Camp Funston couldn't have imagined where it would go.

Still, it didn't catch the American medical establishment completely by surprise. In past wars, the number of dead due to disease compared to or surpassed the number killed in combat, and most military doctors expected this war to be no different. It was unimaginable that the day might come when fighting epidemic disease wasn't synonymous with fighting a war.

In fact, during wartime, epidemics of micro-organisms that incubated among groups of closely packed, unhealthy soldiers eventually affected the civilian population as well. In addition, doctors and nurses called to the front to treat combat injuries were obviously no longer available to attend to epidemic sufferers, military or civilian.

War planners understood that the likeliest candidate for an epidemic was bacterial pneumonia, because in that era it was the leading cause of death in America every year. But germ theory was just gaining acceptance, and scientists still didn't understand viruses. In fact, bacteria played a role with Spanish flu, too, as bacterial pneumonia and sinus infections were common secondary complications and leading causes of death brought on by the H1N1 Spanish flu virus.

This H1N1 strain is frequently referred to as the Spanish flu even though it neither started in Spain nor peaked there, although Spain did have one of the worst early outbreaks. And the Spanish discussed this strange flu more extensively than many other cultures. They had not been drawn into the war, so they didn't censor their news to manipulate public morale and were able to devote more of their national debate to the topic.

The Spanish flu virus emerged in 1918 the same way all variations on the influenza virus do. The flu virus spread from person to person, probably in very cramped quarters, via airborne respiratory secretions, the familiar coughing and sneezing of any respiratory infection. The first wave of infections was relatively mild. Though hundreds of men at Camp Funston became ill, only thirty-eight died of pneumonia. Since this flu was not yet the terrifying killer it would become, it didn't garner much attention. Because of that, it may have spread somewhat undetected among American troops preparing to leave for Europe.

It seems these GIs must have brought it with them from home, because by April it had appeared in Western Europe. It spread quickly across the continent, reaching Poland by the summer.

By August, the H1N1 strain appeared to have become more lethal. It has been speculated that after passing once around the world, it must have mutated into something more effective at reaching deep into the lungs of its victims, perhaps turning the immune systems of young and healthy victims against them as they choked on copious secretions. The virus spread more and more quickly, dashing around the globe to become a true pandemic. In the end, it swept across Europe and North America, down through Latin America, into Asia and Africa, and even to the most remote islands on the globe.

To take just one example of its fury in an American military facility, 1 reported infection at Camp Devens, Massachusetts, became 6,674 cases in only six days. By 1919, the flu had killed a total of at least 550,000 Americans and perhaps as many as 50 million or more across the rest of the world, wreaking the most havoc in India, where it killed 17 million people alone.

The Spanish flu was easily the most destructive influenza outbreak in history. As has been widely reported, more United States soldiers died from the Spanish flu during World War I than from the war itself.

How a flu pandemic could start

It is far more likely that the Spanish flu began in Asia or India than among the poultry population in Kansas. In the 1990s, the H1N1virus, which had been preserved from several victims, was studied in the laboratory and determinations were made about what had happened back in 1918. H1N1 most likely started out in waterfowl like most influenza A viruses and then infected poultry before mutating to a form that could easily infect humans. There is no record of a large outbreak in birds, and it is reasonable to conclude that this virus, so deadly to humans after it mutated, was not that deadly to birds beforehand.

Poultry, including chickens and turkeys, are bred for all sorts of characteristics, mostly related to the amount and quality of meat each bird can produce. Wildfowl, however, are concerned only with survival, and as one might expect, they are more resistant to diseases, including influenza infections, than their domestic counterparts.

All birds are susceptible to avian influenza, although some species are more resistant than others. In birds, different strains of flu can cause any range of symptoms from mild illness to a highly contagious and rapidly fatal disease. Strains with a sudden onset, severe illness, and rapid death are called highly pathogenic avian influenza.

Migratory waterfowl, especially ducks, are the natural reservoir of the avian influenza virus. Since no one is checking or treating them for diseases, viruses (especially nonfatal ones) spread unchecked throughout their population. While birds make antibodies to protect them against flu, the influenza virus continues to adapt and may change rapidly. These mutations sometimes become new forms of the virus, in a process known as antigenic drift.

Most influenza epidemics occur when ducks or geese with a new strain of virus come into contact with poultry. Domestic poultry are carefully monitored for influenza, even the mildest cases, because their lower tolerance means one infection can quickly become a highly fatal epidemic. This is especially true for H5 or H7 varieties of avian flu, which tend to be the most deadly among birds.

If a mutation occurs to allow an influenza A to pass among humans, it can become our yearly flu strain. (Influenza B occurs natively in humans, but influenza A has to mutate first.) Antigenic drift keeps scientists and vaccine makers on their toes, trying to match the yearly vaccine with the yearly antigenic variety of human flu.

Luckily for us, the barrier between birds and people is a species barrier, and it is much harder for a bird flu to cross to humans than from one type of bird to another. There are therefore thousands of bird flus that never make the jump. For a bird flu subtype to become a true human virus, one that can be passed from person to person, requires antigenic drift or a more unusual process where bird and human viruses merge, known as antigenic shift.

Theoretically, this merging or shifting of viral particles could happen in the body of a person carrying a human flu who also became infected simultaneously with a bird flu. However, most experts believe these shifts are much more common among pigs.

Pigs make an excellent mixing bowl for influenza because they are susceptible to both bird and mammal varieties. A pig infected with both a human and a bird virus at the same time can develop a hybrid. But what sort of hybrid is very difficult to predict. Remember Vincent Price in *The Fly*? He went into a molecule mixer with an unnoticed fly and came out a monstrous killer with a fly's head and a human body. Meanwhile, somewhere out in the garden was a fly body with a human head that became the helpless victim of a spider. One message from this is that there is simply no controlling or predicting genetics. Similarly, if a hybrid flu bug manages to connect the deadly aspects of a bird bug with the "legs" of a human flu, it could become a monstrous human killer. However, this new subtype, being a mix of the two, could exhibit completely different qualities than the originals. A deadly bird flu could become a mild human flu. A mild bird flu could become a deadly human one.

Remember the famous, and probably fictional, story of the time Albert Einstein and Marilyn Monroe supposedly met. She was reported to have said to him, "Imagine if we got together and had kids with my looks and your brains." And he supposedly replied, "Yes, but imagine if the kids had my looks and your brains." The same problem applies to viruses as well.

A major human influenza A pandemic—which could start as a mutated bird or pig virus—seems to occur, on average, three to four times each century. But no one can be certain when that pandemic will happen, or which virus will be involved.

Fortunately, the last three pandemics in the United States have been getting progressively milder: from over 500,000 dead in 1918 to between 50,000 and 100,000 in 1957 to between 25,000 and 50,000 in 1968. Is this a coincidence, or is it the effects of modern medicine in combating the flu?

Avian outbreaks

Since 1959, the world has seen twenty-one new strains of avian influenza viruses, mostly in Europe and the Americas, not in Asia. Of these new strains, only five spread to numerous chicken farms and only one of those spread to other countries.

Even though these outbreaks were more limited and less formidable than H5N1 has become, it took a significant effort to control them in birds. Even well-managed, well-resourced efforts can take as long as two years to curb an outbreak of a new avian flu strain.

Quarantining farms and destroying exposed flocks has become the standard, primary measure for combating the spread of virus among birds. However, since the highly pathogenic viruses can survive long periods in the environment, especially in low temperatures, farmers need to closely disinfect any farm equipment, cages, or clothing that may have become contaminated.

The last large-scale outbreak of highly pathogenic avian influenza in the United States took place in 1983 in Pennsylvania. This strain took two years to control. More than 17 million birds were destroyed, at a direct cost of $62 million, with an estimated related cost of $250 million. If you ponder how complicated and expensive this was for a developed nation with a less pernicious strain of flu, you begin to understand the monumental economic challenge facing Asia today.

The last major international outbreak among poultry (the H5N2 strain) occurred in Mexico in 1995. Although it has been brought under control, despite years of intense efforts and more than 2 billion doses of vaccines administered, the H5N2 subtype has yet to be eradicated.

Flu pandemics in humans

Slowing the rate of infection has more of an impact on reducing the death toll from a pandemic than on curing those who are infected. Fortunately for our collective survival, most viruses, as they mutate, become good at either spreading or killing, but not both. A virus that is easily and quickly spread tends not to be deadly. People who get only slightly sick are more likely to go about their daily life, spreading the disease everywhere they go. Rhinoviruses, which cause the common cold, are a good example of this. Almost everyone who comes in contact with the virus contracts it, but the symptoms are so mild that people decline to rest and instead go around spreading infection.

Whereas a virus that causes strong symptoms tends to be much slower in spreading. The symptoms themselves keep the patients at home. An example is the so-called stomach virus (norovirus). Once a localized outbreak starts, usually from food handling, it quickly burns out, as most of those infected stay confined to their beds and bathrooms with nausea, vomiting, and diarrhea. While noroviruses are not deadly, and are actually quite common, the short period from exposure to severe symptoms is quick enough to slow its spread.

A pandemic needs to find just the right balance between the two. It must spread quickly, but also be deadly enough to claim a large number of victims. Even the virus of 1918 killed only perhaps one in forty of those infected, but it made up for that by infecting hundreds of millions of people in a very short amount of time.

After the Spanish flu, the next global pandemic was much milder. Advances in public health, medicine, and epidemiology may have been the reason.

The Asian flu was first identified in 1957. Thanks to the new virology of the time, this strain (H2N2) was identified immediately, and a vaccine went intro production by late May 1957. Within a few months, a limited supply of vaccine became available. The virus was, in fact, a repeat performer from the prior century, so few were still alive who had immunity to it.

As the infection spread through the fall, the rates of infection were highest among school children, young adults, and pregnant women, but the elderly had the highest rates of death. The pandemic peaked in midwinter. Close to a million people died globally, with 69,800 people dying in the United States—about double a normal flu year.

The most recent influenza pandemic came when the H3N2 strain appeared, first detected in Hong Kong in 1968 and now commonly referred to as the Hong Kong flu. It spread to the United States that fall, again peaking in winter, and again claiming its highest rate of victims among the elderly.

The Hong Kong flu continued the trend of weaker and weaker pandemics, with only 33,800 American deaths. This pandemic was heading for its peak just as the holidays came, and may have been slowed as much by the closing of virus-spreading classrooms as by the new technologies.

Subtype H5N1 rare human cases

When an apparent new strain of avian flu appeared in Hong Kong in 1997, quick action was taken. Hong Kong's entire poultry population, around 1.5 million birds, were slaughtered, and many experts believed this aggressive culling prevented a wider pandemic.

Of some concern at the time was the fact that eighteen humans had become infected with the virus and six had died. Reassuring was the fact that each of these patients had become infected from direct contact with an infected bird, not an infected person.

International attention to bird flus then shifted to the Netherlands, where a different strain of influenza (H7N7) began killing poultry. It spread across over eight hundred farms before culling brought it under control. Over 11 million chickens were killed. Eighty-three people contracted the disease, but with the help of Tamiflu and the fact that this virus wasn't that deadly to humans, only one died.

Up to the end of 2003, H5N1 was considered a rare disease. But in mid-December of 2003 it reappeared in the Republic of Korea. By January 2004, Vietnam and Thailand both reported human cases of H5N1. In Japan, it appeared in chickens, the first time that country experienced a bird flu since 1925. In early 2004, it also turned up on a duck farm in China.

In August 2004, Chinese scientists announced that they had found H5N1 in pigs, heightening global concerns about the spread to humans, since pigs are the ideal "mixing vessel" for avian and human influenza. The virus had spread though much of Southeast Asia, despite the culling over 100 million chickens.

By October 2004, forty-four people in those countries had become infected from contact with infected birds, of whom thirty-two had died. As I will discuss in a later chapter, many more may have been exposed but not gotten sick, so the exact death rate of the rare H5N1 case in humans isn't known.

World Health Organization officials publicly stated their concerns that this virus could be the source of the next flu pandemic. They started international meetings with governments, doctors, and drug manufacturers to determine the world's level of preparedness.

In the first few weeks of 2005, thirteen Vietnamese citizens contracted H5N1 and twelve of them died. By May, sporadic cases of people dying of bird flu had occurred in several Asian countries. And Indonesia reported finding the virus in pigs.

By the end of August, the Philippines, the last Asian country without the disease, reported an outbreak in ducks and an unconfirmed case in a human. Russia, Tibet, and Kazakhstan also confirmed several cases in poultry. The virus seemed to be spreading from direct contact between wild, migratory waterfowl and domestic poultry. As fall approached, confirmed cases of the strain had spread to Romania, Greece, and Turkey.

In early December 2005, twenty-five hundred domestic birds died in Ukraine, in a remote region of the Crimean Peninsula. But Ukraine's top veterinary surgeon, Petro Verbytsky, urged people to focus on the coming human flu season rather than on bird flu. "The question now is that of dealing with a different sort of [human] flu," he said. "There is 1,000 times less chance of becoming ill from bird flu than there is from tuberculosis."

Actually, even in Ukraine, where bird flu now existed, the chances of becoming ill and dying from tuberculosis were many thousand times greater than dying from bird flu.

Aggressive culling remains the first line of action in response to finding newly infected birds. Large commercial farmers have been cooperative despite a loss of income. They understand the issue well and have trained workers to complete the culling. They use protective equipment and even Tamiflu for those workers who are most exposed.

Despite this, many of the Asian countries currently fighting the outbreak have had trouble controlling the spread of the disease in birds. This is because many of the owners of the birds are poor farmers, who rely heavily on their small stock to survive. In several of the affected countries, as much as of 80 percent of the total poultry production comes from small farms or even backyards. In China alone, as many as 7 billion chickens are thought to be living on small farms, in close proximity to humans, domestic animals, and, perhaps most dangerously, pigs. H5N1 mutates rapidly and already has a documented propensity to acquire genes from viruses infecting other animal species.

Recently, the bird flu vaccine has been added to the equation, and it can be effective together with culling to get H5N1 under control. China has already vaccinated 20 million birds, with many millions more to come.

Many officials tracking the proliferation are concerned that the reluctance shown by small farmers to kill their entire flock may well also translate into a reluctance to report potential infections at all. In addition, the preventative measures are difficult for small farmers to undertake. Many of them have trouble creating the quarantined, environmentally controlled holding area necessary to keep their birds away from other birds, livestock, insects, and rodents. These steps are absolutely necessary, because birds that don't die secrete virus for at least ten days, orally and in their feces.

The lack of experience with controlling outbreaks and running successful culling operations is taking its toll. Sometimes officials announce a process complete and an area cleared of infection, only to see more eruptions of disease. It is during these times that officials are the most concerned, when it appears that the process for culling, disinfection, vaccination, and continued detection is simply not working.

Pandemic trends

When a pandemic does occur, and an influenza A that we haven't seen before switches to humans, the bulk of the deaths have always been among those in developing countries. An underdeveloped public health system, lack of adequate medical care, and lack of effective means to spread knowledge and gain the cooperation of those at risk are the essential ingredients of a high death toll.

At the same time, looking at the history of influenza pandemics, there is a positive trend. In industrialized nations, especially the United States, the interval between pandemics is growing longer, the spread of the disease is becoming slower, and the final mortality count is getting smaller.

INFLUENZA A EVOLUTION IN HUMANS

Year	Strain	Development
1874	H3N8	
1890	H2N2	Pandemic
1902	H3N2	
1918	H1N1	Pandemic
1933	H1N1	First strains isolated
1947	H1N1	Variation detected
1957	H2N2	Asian flu
1968	H3N2	Hong Kong flu

3

SPANISH FLU VERSUS
SWINE FLU

As even the most casual bird flu followers must know by now, back in 1918 an influenza virus killed—by many estimates—more than 50 million people. As I've mentioned, it was the most devastating pandemic in recorded history, and almost every article on bird flu makes reference to it. During the outbreak, more people died of influenza in a single year than in the four years of the bubonic plague from 1347 to 1351. Known as the Spanish flu or La Grippe, the 1918 flu famously killed more people than died in battle during all of World War I.

Ever since then, there have been three public reactions to avian influenza. The first is denial. For years before 2004, newspapers would stick any coverage they had about Asian bird flus deep in the unread pages of the international section. This reaction worried the public health community because there are thousands of avian flu bugs and several do mutate sufficiently to pass routinely human to human and cause our yearly flu. The yearly flu, though not pandemic (involving multiple communities at once), is deadly enough to kill on average thirty-six thousand people in the United States every year and hospitalize approximately two hundred thousand.

The second reaction to the ghost of the 1918 killer flu is hysteria, or emotional forecasting based on no real information that this is going to be the year that the Spanish flu—or worse—returns. The reincarnation in this case has been designated the H5N1 virus.

The hysteria in the United States has been fueled in part by the disaster of Hurricane Katrina. Fearmongers, leaders, and serious public health experts alike have pointed to the lack of preparation and poor reaction to this hurricane as justification for concern about avian influenza. We were unprepared for one major disaster, the reasoning goes, and avian influenza is another major disaster waiting to happen. We seem no better prepared for pandemic flu. The problem with this direct parallel is that the levees in New Orleans were faulty and the effects of the hurricane were a likely scenario. The fact that the potential hurricane that New Orleans officials have been ignoring for decades finally hit this year does not rationally predict that a massive pandemic from bird flu will hit this year as well.

In fact, the specter of the Spanish flu has fueled previous overreactions. The most prominent example occurred in 1976, when the swine flu made the jump from birds to pigs to humans. This outbreak has many parallels with today's concern with the H5N1 bird flu, but it rarely gets treated that way in the media. That's because it never did

SPANISH FLU VERSUS SWINE FLU

wipe out millions as was feared, dead-ending instead. The fear in 1976 was so great that over 40 million were vaccinated in a month in the United States using a hastily made vaccine that appears to have caused more than a thousand cases of Guillain-Barré syndrome, a form of ascending paralysis from which some people never recover.

The third reaction to the ghost of 1918 is the most reasoned one, somewhere in the unexplored middle ground between denial and hysteria, and takes into account both the fact that another pandemic is inevitable and that its magnitude and its timing are unknown. In any case, the current plan of protection for a worst-case scenario is woefully inadequate. Some scientists, public health officials, and journalists have set about informing the public with the expressed goal that shining a spotlight on this potential risk of avian influenza will provoke an allotment of resources designed to protect us for any outbreak. This plan must contain some allowance for a worst-case scenario (stockpiles of vaccines and antiviral drugs) while at the same time working to improve the hospital and public health infrastructure on the federal, state, and local levels. Even if it's not likely to arrive this winter, if a devastating pandemic does occur, we can be ready for it.

A key feature of a well-thought-out plan would include a focus on upgrading the method used to make our vaccines by using genetic technology and cell culture so that, if necessary, millions of doses of a safely manufactured vaccine could be made in a hurry.

Such a program would put us far ahead of where the medical world was in 1918 when medical science was so backward that doctors reacting to the outbreak of the Spanish flu thought it must be caused by bacteria.

The blue death

In the fall of 1918, around the globe, perhaps beginning in the Indian army, perhaps beginning in the American army, an infection took hold that was at first perceived to be no more than a cold. However, as it spread from America through Europe, it became more deadly. It quickly killed many who lived in the poor conditions of the combat trenches, but far more than that, it sped around the globe, killing tens of millions of people, including an estimated 17 million in India, where it did most of its damage.

But few countries were spared. Surprisingly, the flu was most deadly for young adults, between the ages of twenty and forty, rather than the very young and the elderly, whom most flus affect. Some experts have postulated in retrospect that it was the heightened immune response that healthy people can muster that somehow did them in. Their lungs may have filled up with infection-fighting secretions they couldn't clear. Most experts agree that the most common cause of death was pneumonia and respiratory failure. Most likely, the pneumonia was due to a secondary bacterial pneumonia for which there were no antibiotic treatments available at the time. For those who survived, the virus also appears to have caused neurological side effects in many patients, including an inflammation of the brain (encephalopathy), which often led to permanent disabilities.

The flu also brought out many other chronic conditions such as heart disease, asthma, and diabetes, for which there were no ready treatments.

In the end, the Spanish flu infected at least 28 percent of all Americans, and at least 675,000 died, ten times as many as in the Great War. Half of the American soldiers who died in Europe died from influenza rather than from combat.

As noted in the *Journal of the American Medical Association*'s final edition of 1918: "1918 has gone: a year momentous as the termination of the most cruel war in the annals of the human race; a year which marked, the end at least for a time, of man's destruction of man; unfortunately a year in which developed a most fatal infectious disease causing the death of hundreds of thousands of human beings. Medical science for four and one-half years devoted itself to putting men on the firing line and keeping them there. Now it must turn with its whole might to combating the greatest enemy of all: infectious disease."

Even with the Spanish flu, the worst of all plagues, most victims recovered, and their experience generally was a more intense version of the expected weeklong course of fever, aches, chills, and nausea that characterized all influenza. But a substantial minority endured much worse. They were exhausted, with earaches, headaches, high fever, and difficult breathing.

Doctors with little experience diagnosing viruses (they still didn't really know what a virus was) often confused the Spanish flu with a cold until the patients were very sick.

Some patients died rapidly, sometimes overnight. They turned cyanotic (meaning they turned blue), struggled for air, and were choked by their blood-tinged secretions. As the disease progressed and pneumonia set in, they began to bleed profusely—from the nose, the ears, and the mouth. Some still recovered. But if cyanosis appeared, physicians treated patients as terminal. Autopsies would show a disease that ravaged almost every internal organ.

The pandemic circled the globe, often following trade routes and shipping lines. Outbreaks coursed through North America, Europe, Asia, Brazil, and the South Pacific. Soldiers spread it to far lands on ships. The Committee on Atmosphere and Man concluded in 1923 that humidity was a factor in the spread of the disease.

The origin of the Spanish flu is not known, although the current prevailing theory is that it started in China. In the spring of 1918 it first arrived in the United States in Kansas and in U.S. military camps, where it wasn't acknowledged initially—the focus instead being on the winding down of the war.

The war brought a second wave of the virus back in September, and by then it appeared much more deadly, perhaps because of further mutations to the viral structure, first arriving in Boston in late August, and with two hundred thousand dying of it in October alone. The United States Public Health Service (USPHS) was in charge of coordinating care among the states, but the wartime shortage of doctors, and especially nurses, made this care very difficult to deliver on a consistent basis. Congress appropriated $1 million to the USPHS, but didn't appropriate funds specifically for influenza research. The USPHS did appoint a director for influenza in each state but wasn't effective in coordinating care. People often died of dehydration, starvation, and poor care, rather than the flu itself. Disorganization and lack of solid disseminated information contributed to the problem. Doctors, with no vaccines or treatments available and a poor understanding of the disease, turned desperate, even using unproven nonviral-based vaccines (often targeting some imagined bacteria). This was at a time when most doctors had been taught in medical school that bleeding patients was the best known cure for pneumonia. Doctors urged cities to quarantine the sick and restrict attendance at public gatherings, but wartime rallies and draft registrations supervened.

Urban conditions were crowded, poorly ventilated, and filthy—conducive to the spread of disease. Schools, cinemas, churches, and public meeting houses were supposed to be closed, and attempts were made to force infected patients into hospital wards, but many of these ordinances were ignored by people who didn't realize the danger they were in. Many cities refused to shut their public transit systems until hundreds of sick transit workers forced them to do so. Boston ignored the epidemic initially, because of the city's seeming good health, and the country only began to pay attention in late September, when the disease had already spread to places as far away from Boston as Seattle.

Entire Navy fleets were sick with the disease and were too ill to fight, and military hospitals, already overcome with the war wounded (including burns from mustard gas), were unequipped to treat the flu. Soldiers lived and traveled in cramped conditions conducive to the spread of the virus.

On top of this, there was a shortage of physicians and nurses. Medical personnel discovered that having potentially infected people wear a surgical mask helped limit the spread of infection—until they ran out of gauze to make surgical masks. They understood that administering oxygen to patients in distress was helpful, but they didn't have the means to administer it to even a small percentage of the patients who needed it. They understood that overcrowding soldiers into barracks and packing patients wall to wall in hospitals were making things worse, but they had no alternative. The differences between the resources available to us today and those available a century ago are staggering.

The nation even experienced a shortage of coffins and grave diggers. Funerals were limited to fifteen minutes. Bodies piled up, as they had during the bubonic plague of the fourteenth century, in hospitals, in carts, in homes, in hallways, in the streets.

The Red Cross responded to the nursing shortage by asking for volunteers and by creating the National Committee on Influenza. Emergency hospitals were created to take in those sick with influenza as well as those arriving sick from overseas. With one quarter of the United States and one fifth of the world infected, it was impossible to escape from it, though the wealthy and the famous were fairly successful at sequestering themselves. But even President Woodrow Wilson caught influenza in early 1919, while negotiating the Treaty of Versailles.

Scientists, using the recently accepted germ theory, worked unsuccessfully on a vaccine. Public health officials, capitalizing on restrictions already in place for the war, tried to restrict movements between U.S. cities. Railroads wouldn't accept passengers without signed documentation attesting to no infection. But overall, the public health response was characterized by confusion, disorganization, ineffectiveness, and edicts that weren't followed.

And then, as quickly as it had come, in 1919, perhaps aided by the coming of spring, when flu viruses traditionally fail to thrive, the Spanish flu died out.

After 1918, research identified the virus that causes influenza as well as the bacteria-like pneumonia that causes its secondary, life-threatening complications. Public health officials are far better these days than in 1918 at public education and promoting public co-operation. One can only speculate about what would have happened in 1918 if they had available to them even a tenth of the technology and methods that we have today.

Still, the world is much more densely populated, and air travel allows people to travel (and potentially spread disease) to far-off places in only a matter of hours. But while a plane covers a lot ground very quickly, a 1918 military ship in the middle of the high seas, densely packed with exhausted young men eating and sleeping in close quarters, makes for a better environment to grow and spread a virus.

As hard as it is to make direct comparisons between 1918 and the present, it's easier to make comparisons with the swine flu, which occurred just thirty years ago.

1976

On February 5, 1976, nineteen-year-old Private David Lewis of Massachusetts told his drill instructor at Fort Dix that he felt tired and weak. Nevertheless, he participated in a training hike and within twenty-four hours he was dead. Two weeks after his death, health officials, calling Lewis the "index case" and having isolated five hundred other cases of what they called "swine flu" in other recruits who hadn't gotten sick and four who had, disclosed to the American public that there was concern about a possible epidemic. Public panic ensued, as health officials reasoned that any flu that was able to reach so many people so fast was capable of becoming a worldwide plague.

With the specter of 1918 firmly in their minds, public health officials quickly considered the possibility of mass inoculations before the next flu season, worrying that as in 1918 the flu virus might get stronger by its second season, or "wave."

Some experts maintain that this was a great example of America's public health community acting in advance of what could easily have been a new plague. At the time, the Spanish flu was wrongly understood to have developed from exposure to pigs, as swine flu clearly had. The accepted theory was that bird flus and human flus comingle in pigs and that the required mutation necessary to give a bird flu "human legs" occurs most easily by that exchange of genetic material in a pig's blood (antigenic shift). This theory is still believed today to be a likely method of transmitting many animal flu viruses to humans. In fact, a study published online by *Clinical Infectious Diseases* on November 22, 2005, and sponsored by the National Institutes of Allergies and Infectious Diseases is the latest research to show that frequent exposure to swine flu viruses leads to seroconversion (making antibodies) in food handlers and pig farmers.

Back in 1976, operating on the assumption that the swine flu virus that had been discovered was very similar to the 1918 flu bug, public health officials, leaders, and subsequently the public were all worried. No one knew how the swine flu had gotten to Fort Dix, but all were concerned that it could spread rapidly from there.

Weeks after Private Lewis died, doctors from the Centers for Disease Control, including the director, Dr. David Spencer, the sagacious polio vaccine inventors Salk and Sabin, and other officials met in Washington, D.C., to decide what to do. They were concerned about swine flu, but they were also concerned that attempts to rapidly immunize the public would interrupt work on many other diseases. They could only imagine, however, the complaints doctors would face if an epidemic broke out and vaccines weren't ready. At the same time, they couldn't help wondering what would happen if everyone was inoculated for a plague that didn't happen.

By March 1976, Dr. Spencer had lined up most of the medical establishment behind his plan to ask the president for $135 million to mass vaccinate the country.

But there may have been more to it than simple medical concerns. It may also have been political. In his book *Pure Politics and Impure Science*, Arthur M. Silverstein suggests that presidential politics played a heavy role in this decision, as President Gerald Ford, up for re-election and under the influence of America's big drug manufacturers, wanted to be seen as a hero.

On March 24, the day after a surprise loss to Ronald Reagan in the North Carolina Republican primary, Ford made his announcement to the public and prepared to take this battle to Congress. Meanwhile, the drug makers were insisting that the government take liability for any harmful side effects from a hastily made vaccine. Congressional hearings stretched on into the early summer, with some doubting Thomases (I'm not the first doctor, clearly, to have doubts) pointing out that swine flu hadn't extended beyond Fort Dix in its "first wave."

Ultimately, the president and his experts prevailed, and on August 12, 1976, Congress approved the funding. Dr. W. Delano Meriwether of the Department of Health, Education and Welfare, a thirty-three-year-old physician and world-class sprinter, was put in charge of the project and given until the end of the year to inoculate all 220 million Americans against swine flu.

When insurance companies refused to provide coverage to the vaccine manufacturers, the government finally agreed to accept liability for claims of adverse events. This obstacle having been cleared, the National Influenza Immunization Program (NIIP) officially started in October 1976.

By October 1 the serum was ready, and the public health system had organized doctors, nurses, and para-professionals to give out the shots. But within days, several people who had taken the shot fell seriously ill. Three elderly people in Pennsylvania had their shots and died just a few hours later of heart attacks, which caused the program to be immediately suspended in that state.

Other states pressed on, even as more reports of adverse side effects came out.

The number of vaccinations given each week increased rapidly from less than 1 million in early October to more than 4 million in the later weeks of the month, and reached a peak of more than 6 million doses a week by the middle of November 1976. The NIIP was unique in the annals of epidemiology: an organized surveillance effort was in place from the very beginning, and over 40 million people were vaccinated during the short time the NIIP was in effect. However, on December 16, 1976, the NIIP was suspended following reports from more than ten states of Guillain-Barré syndrome (GBS) in vaccinees. By January 1977, more than five hundred cases of GBS had been reported, with twenty-five deaths. The government suspended the program. Millions of dollars in lawsuits followed.

The swine flu never came

One question you regularly hear in the media is, could we react to a pandemic if we needed to? In 1976, our public health officials pulled off an astonishing public health feat to counter what they thought was an emerging plague based on 1918 fears. But, rather than learn from this event now, we leave it buried in history. Public health officials both then and now speak with an apparent certainty that does not always reflect the amount of speculation involved. Swine flu showed not only that you can rush to judgment, wasting time and money ramping up for a worst-case scenario that never comes, but that in doing so, there may also be significant costs to people's health.

The swine flu scare helped foster cynicism and distrust of federal policy makers and health officials. But Joseph Califano, who subsequently became secretary of the Department of Health, Education and Welfare under President Carter, continued to maintain that doctors had had no choice but to err on the side of caution, and should do so again if faced with the threat of another killer plague with the potential to kill millions.

What is Guillain-Barré Syndrome?

Back in 1976, the rushed swine flu vaccination program caused measurable medical damage.

Guillain-Barré syndrome (GBS) is a fairly uncommon neurologic disorder characterized by sudden muscular weakness, especially in the hands and feet, though in more severe cases the muscles of breathing are involved. Symptoms of paralysis may progress for up to ten days. Patients often improve, and recovery tends to occur within three months. Some unusual cases have been difficult to diagnose.

The exact cause of GBS remains unknown. It was always believed to be due to a virus, but more recently it has been seen as an immunological reaction to an invading agent (including virus particles).

For the first time ever, in the swine flu vaccination program, a nationwide surveillance system was established to evaluate illnesses that might be due to the vaccination. The network was coordinated by the CDC with state and local mandatory participation. A registration consent form had to be signed by all vaccinees. Any illness serious enough to cause hospitalization had to be telephoned in to the CDC.

In August 1977 the results were released to the public. Alexander Langmuir, director of the epidemiology branch of the National Communicable Disease Center in Atlanta, presented a preliminary report in 1979. Based on the weekly numbers of vaccinations, a comparison of observed with expected cases showed that the relative risk of acquiring GBS during the six weeks after vaccination was about ten times the expectation. Langmuir concluded that the vaccine contained a "trigger element" leading to GBS in one in one hundred thousand of those who received the vaccine.

Also in 1979, Dr. Lawrence Schonberger and his collaborators at the CDC presented an additional analysis of the national surveillance data of cases. A total of 1,098 cases of GBS had been reported to the CDC during the four months under investigation in 1976. (There are no doubt many more cases that weren't reported.) Subsequently, lawsuits led to re-evaluation of the cases by a panel formed by Langmuir. The apparent association between the vaccine and the development of GBS was again confirmed.

Soon after the publication of this study, Nathan Mantel, at the time a professor of statistics at George Washington University, released criticisms suggesting that the number of cases that occurred late had been underreported by both Langmuir and Schonberger and that more compensation should have been considered. However, subsequent studies in Michigan and Ohio in 1984 showed that the main risk period had really been six weeks after vaccination, as had been reported.

In a key finding, both Schonberger and Langmuir had discovered that among cases of GBS, those in the vaccinated group had a much lower incidence of another explanation for the GBS, namely an acute viral-type illness. The "trigger element" in 1976 could have been one of the proteins from the virus used to make the vaccine. Luckily, subsequent flu vaccines have not shown an increased incidence of GBS (except for a possible slight increase in 1992 and 1993).

A Harvard study in 1997 by Elissa Laitin and Elise Pelletier—reviewing all the prior studies—concluded that there is strong evidence to show a causal link between the swine flu vaccine and GBS. This conclusion is possible thanks to the well-organized surveillance effort in 1976, a key tool of epidemiology.

At the same time, many cases probably went unrecognized or unreported at the time. I received this recent correspondence, for example. "I was stationed at Fort Dix in early 1976 as a fresh young recruit during the swine flu period. We were vaccinated with a vaccine. I become very ill during this period and was hospitalized at the main base hospital. Please, I was hoping you could provide me with the name of the condition or disease which causes a type of paralysis."

One positive outcome of the swine flu vaccine/GBS disaster was the development of the National Vaccine Injury Compensation Program in 1988, which compensates people for vaccine-related injuries or death.

My goal in including this section in this book is not to replace the obsessive fear of a bird flu with the fear of a vaccine, hoping that one will cancel the other out, as it did in 2002 when a nonexistent disease—smallpox—created unrealistic fears until these were replaced by fears of the antiquated live virus vaccine that was being hauled out of mothballs to treat it.

Instead, the swine flu lesson is more one about cost and benefit. Prevention is always a wise consideration, but it isn't without risk. The ghosts of 1918 can certainly teach valuable lessons, but they can also help provoke a hasty reaction to a new virus that can itself cause harm while those in charge guard unthinkingly against a worst-case scenario.

Careful consideration should always be given to the science on all sides. In the case of swine flu, there simply wasn't enough scientific evidence to back the conviction that many officials had that a giant pandemic was imminent. No one wanted to admit that at that point in time they were speculating about the 1918 virus and applying that speculation to the 1976 swine flu, a trend that has passed from them on to us.

2006

In 2006, our scientists still believe that the pig can commingle bird and human flu viruses and cause an antigenic shift that may lead to the next flu pandemic. But back in 1976, it was also believed that the Spanish flu of 1918 picked up its essential mutation in pigs, a contention that has since been challenged by studying the structure of the 1918 molecule itself. Studies over the past ten years have shown that the 1918 H1N1 influenza A virus made the jump directly from birds to humans, which has prompted the recent speculation that the current H5N1 killer bird virus is about to do the same.

But speculation is not science. And science is an on-going series of observations, not an assertion that is blindly adhered to (such as "The world is flat") despite corrective facts. In 1976, such a course correction should have been made when the supposed "first wave" of the outbreak that was to approximate the one of 1918 never made it out of Fort Dix. Ignoring that important fact showed strong conviction, but it wasn't good science.

Now in 2006, where we again face an inflamed situation, with plans afoot to ramp up vaccine production against a virus that doesn't yet threaten us, and with our vaccine manufacturers again asking for a free pass against liability, we have to incorporate the lessons of 1976 as well as those of 1918.

The lessons of 1918 are best learned when contrasted with the massive fear-driven reaction in 1976. The fact that swine flu never became an epidemic is not the point. Officials were afraid of being unprepared, and perhaps they made the wrong choice, though it seemed reasonable to many at the time. But in 2006, we have no excuse. We have the results of both 1918 and 1976 to inform us. We could make the public debate about whether this current bird flu is potentially more like Spanish flu or swine flu. Instead, we turn the debate all the way to the dark side, speculating about whether this unmutated virus is as bad as Spanish flu, or even worse.

A major problem in 1918 was that the country wasn't focused on public health and instead continued to rely on old solutions that didn't work. It is not reasonable to simply apply the Spanish flu experience to today's world, which is more overcrowded and easily traveled but also has the antibiotics, steroids, heart and diabetes medication, sanitation, and public health that 1918 didn't have. Despite these essential differences, by the time 1976 rolled around, a lot of the facts had been forgotten and 1918 became a code word for lack of preparation. We invoked 1918 and instantly reacted to whatever threat we thought we faced.

In 2006, there is concern about bird flu, but there is no real imminence, and 1976-style panic is not productive or realistic. Preparation for some pandemic, not necessarily H5N1, is a long-term issue that involves improving hospital and emergency responder readiness as well as upgrading how we make vaccines—the use of technology, cell culture, and genetic engineering, all technologies we now have and use routinely for other vaccines.

4

A BIRD'S-EYE VIEW

I t occurs to me that our tendency to look at the risks of avian influenza from an entirely human medical perspective may be a crucial mistake. Whenever I see our top health officials, Drs. Anthony Fauci, Julie Gerberding, Michael Osterholm, and Mike Leavitt, on TV answering questions about bird flu, I think, What about the veterinarians? After all, avian influenza is a bird disease; its natural reservoir is waterfowl, not man. Who better to analyze and make predictions than the animal doctors who study birds? Even better than bird experts, how about bird experts who are experts in infectious diseases among birds?

I spoke with Elizabeth Krushinskie, D.V.M., Ph.D., and vice president of Food Safety and Production Programs at the U.S. Poultry and Egg Association. She acknowledged at the outset her potential bias—her livelihood is in commercial agriculture—but considering that the entire poultry industry is at risk not only from bird flu but even more so from irrational fear of bird flu, her bias seems relevant.

I also spoke with David Swayne, D.V.M., Ph.D., and director of the Southeast Poultry Research Lab division of the USDA, as well as Dr. Ron De Haven, D.V.M. and chief administrator for animal and plant health at the USDA. Dr. Swayne's answers to my questions were sent by e-mail and were preapproved by the communications division of the USDA because of the sensitive nature of his work and of the topic itself. Dr. Swayne is generally considered to be one of the world's top experts on avian influenza.

Dr. Krushinskie agreed that fear is now the prevailing virus, not avian flu. She said, "Fear is causing a great amount of poultry damage in the United States and around the world. For example, poultry consumption in Armenia dropped off 50% without even a single case, because of one case in Turkey [the country]. What can we do?"

Each time the disease spreads to another region of the world, that area's poultry flock is jeopardized more by fear than by H5N1. In October 2005, when a parrot was found to have the disease in Great Britain, poultry consumption in that country dropped 30 percent. In November 2005, when a chicken in Western Canada was found to be infected by a different avian flu bug that is far more benign than the one coursing through Southeast Asia, Japan immediately swore off importation of Canadian poultry, and the United States temporarily refrained from importing chickens from Western Canada.

Imagine what will happen if even a single scraggly

goose in the United States acquires the H5N1 bird flu. Despite the fact that cooking a chicken kills the virus, and that most of our poultry is housed far away from our waterfowl, our poultry industry will crumble instantly as other countries will stop taking our imports, and we Americans will panic further and many of us will stop eating fowl altogether.

Speaking and corresponding with Krushinskie, Swayne, and De Haven, three seasoned veterinarians who have studied and tracked avian influenza throughout their careers, I was able to appreciate the larger context. Bird flu is a disease that resides in waterfowl. The bird flu (influenza A) virus is a small package of DNA that changes a lot, but in the vast majority of cases is non-pathogenic and dead-ends in birds.

As I've mentioned earlier, all influenza virus envelopes contain two essential molecules, a hemagglutinin (with 16 possible varieties) and a neuraminidase (9 varieties). There are 144 different subtypes. The hemagglatinin and the neuraminidase proteins are the facilitators of infection. The neuraminidase molecule cleaves the hemagglutinin in its hinge region, whereupon the virus folds over and is able to attach to the surface of the host cell. When new virus particles are ready to break free of the cell and make the jump to neighboring cells, it is again the neuraminidase enzyme that helps them to do so.

If this is the ordinary course of events for a bird flu, then what turns an avian virus into a ferocious bird killer? This occurs when the virus, chumming through cellular rubble, acquires enough proteins so that it can be cut loose from cells more easily, cleaved not only by its neuraminidases but also by commonly found molecules known as proteases.

These changes make a flu virus more frisky. A hyperactive virus jumping easily from cell to cell is thereby more deadly. But deadly can mean deadly in one species and not in another. Duck proteases, for example, do not work effectively on any avian flu virus no matter how many new proteins it picks up. This is why the duck is the essential reservoir or carrier for bird flu, but usually does not die from it.

Dr. Krushinskie is concerned that we may be overestimating how lethal the H5N1 virus is, thereby increasing our worry unnecessarily. She acknowledges that it is quite lethal in birds, close to 80 percent, although she points out that 99 percent of the bird deaths are the results of human culling as we attempt to control the spread of the disease. In Romania in 2000, for example, every bird was killed in the village when just a few birds were found to have the disease.

Krushinskie and Swayne are both in favor of vaccinating as well as killing birds to control potential outbreaks, but Krushinskie cautioned against vaccinating the entire bird population. "Vaccination is an incomplete strategy for eradicating the disease because it turns a hot fire into a brush fire. It interferes with your surveillance strategy. Remember, those birds that die from the flu or from culling can't spread the disease. Those birds that are nonresponders to a vaccine can still spread it."

Krushinskie (and Swayne) believe that the 50 percent mortality rate in humans could be overstated as well. In 1997 in Hong Kong, where people interact closely with birds in a live bird market, there were sixteen cases of human bird flu and six deaths. But what was not widely reported at the time or since is the fact that thousands were screened in the area and 16 percent were antibody positive, which strongly implies that there is a subclinical or milder form of the disease in humans. It also implies that more people have been exposed to this virus than we realize. Unless a person gets very sick, it may not be reported at all. And if a majority of people who are exposed to the virus don't get sick from it, that would mean that the H5N1 bird flu isn't as lethal to humans as has been reported. Krushinskie feels that we should be continuing to do these sero-surveys now in Asia, whenever a human becomes sick with bird flu, so we can figure out just how deadly (or not) it really is to a human host.

Dr. Krushinskie said, "H5N1 in its current form is far from as deadly in humans as we think. Maybe only .001 percent become sick enough to be a clinical case. All this exposure, and the necessary mutations to allow it to pass from human to human haven't happened." She believes that "H5N1 is probably going to run its course and go away. Outside of Southeast Asia there isn't a single human case. There is no selective pressure to drive it towards humans. It could just as easily move away."

Many experts do not agree with Krushinskie. In fact, a concern of many infectious disease experts is that all this exposure to humans and potentially to human flu viruses increases the chances that one will mutate into a form that can infect us. And in the meantime, H5N1 is not just going away. It continues to move, smoldering and erupting, killing chickens, wild birds, and occasionally a human.

The biggest strategic error, according to Krushinskie, is to focus all of our attention on building a big protection against H5N1 here in the United States in humans rather than fighting it across the seas in birds. Krushinskie describes this phenomenon as "building a big firewall and a moat around your house rather than going across the street to put out a fire before it gets to you."

$2.7 billion of the money proposed by President Bush for pandemic preparation is earmarked to upgrade our vaccine capabilities, which seems a wise idea, but less than $300 million is going to fight the problem in birds. "We've got our eye focused on the wrong end of the telescope," Krushinskie said. "We need to go after the disease where it is occurring today, in birds."

Plan of attack

Dr. Ron De Haven, one of the top administrators at the USDA, is traveling the world these days, meeting with top members of the UN Food and Agriculture Organization, the Organization of International Epizootics, and, on the human side of the equation, the World Health Organization and top members of the World Bank. I caught up with Dr. De Haven on the phone from Rome, where he had just met with these top health officials for birds as well as people.

De Haven has an easygoing manner, the cover for a tireless, committed administrator. His main focus these days is to develop an effective response plan that involves human as well as bird strategies. He is more concerned about the possibility of a large-scale H5N1 human pandemic than Krushinskie is, but he agrees that a primary focus should be "attacking the virus at its source. Reducing and delaying it."

De Haven reviewed the history of pathogenic avian influenza. There had been three outbreaks among birds in 1924, 1925, and 1929, all of which had been extinguished in commercial poultry. He also cited a big outbreak of avian influenza in 1983, leading to 17 million birds being destroyed in Pennsylvania and in the Shenandoah Valley, and one in 2004 in Texas, where a flock of boiler chickens was infected with a pathogenic AI strain (not H5N1) and 6,600 birds were killed.

De Haven acknowledged that no previous influenza outbreak in birds had anywhere near the scope of H5N1. He was focused more on containment at this point than on eradication. He had a budget of $4.4 million for biosecurity outreach, which he acknowledged wasn't completely adequate. "We need top surveillance of people and products. Mislabeled chicken feet on a plane could bring the virus in, though it wouldn't spread it. Unlike the Middle East, we don't have a migratory bird pathway, but a Pacific flyaway bird heading over Siberia could bring it in through Alaska."

The USDA believes there needs to be a heightened alert for smuggled poultry products as well as increased vigilance and surveillance of migratory birds. De Haven explained that the incubation period of the disease in birds is seven to ten days and the USDA routinely employs three rounds of surveillance seven days apart. When asked why we haven't seen bird flu here yet, De Haven emphasized repeatedly that our exposure to Asian migratory birds here in the United States is quite low. Still, asymptomatic ducks or geese could bring H5N1 here via Siberia and Alaska, so vigilance is certainly warranted.

De Haven is now working together with his contemporaries around the world to develop a comprehensive strategy of containment, involving screening, vaccination, and culling. Trained teams go to affected regions and make a country-by-country assessment: do these places have the resources to address the problem? Right now, the main countries being targeted are Indonesia, Vietnam, and China. China has already vaccinated 20 million birds on its own, but De Haven is unable to verify the quality or effectiveness of the vaccine they are using.

Everyone's goal is to reduce the worldwide H5N1 viral load with an aggressive program. De Haven believes that the less virus there is around, the less likely a dreaded human-to-human mutation will occur. At the very least, several species of birds are endangered. De Haven said, "Reducing the virus in birds at worst reduces the chances of a human pandemic significantly. At best, it will be a way to control this virus."

The USDA feels that vaccination can help to make significant headway against the H5N1 problem. De Haven is not as concerned as Krushinskie that too much vaccinating may cause a smoldering effect but not extinguish the fire. The USDA has 40 million bird flu vaccines available, with 30 million more on the way and another 40 million planned for. De Haven says this vaccine offers birds excellent protection and is at least ten times less expensive to make than the human version. Sterility and precautions must still be taken in vaccine manufacture, but certainly not to the same extent that vaccines for humans must be scrutinized. The same manufacturer makes vaccines for all the countries that need it, which ensures some consistency to the vaccine's effect. De Haven works with experts in other countries and with the international organizations to make sure there is enough vaccine and that it is being delivered to appropriate places.

De Haven strikes me as someone who rather than panicking is translating his concern to action, developing a preventative strategy in birds. No one knows whether this virus will ever be a real problem for humans, but all experts agree that it is a big problem for birds. "This is a hot virus," he said. "It has the genetic sequence of a very pathogenic strain. We define pathogenic as a virus that kills six out of ten chicks that are inoculated with it in the laboratory. H5N1 killed ten out of ten chicks."

Q and A with Dr. Swayne

The USDA communications office replied to questions I e-mailed to Dr. David Swayne, one of the world's top research experts on avian influenza in birds. I have edited them only for space and to avoid redundancy. I also asked Dr. Swayne two additional questions that the USDA declined to have him answer—the first was whether we should be doing more sero-testing of humans in the vicinity of an outbreak. The USDA communications office (who were on the whole quite cooperative and responsive) indicated that was too much of a "human" question for him to answer. The second question was what he thinks the chances are of H5N1 mutating to a form that can cause the next human pandemic. The USDA answered that one for him. "The answer is unknown."

Do you agree that far more resources should be used to target H5N1 in the bird population before throwing all our resources into human preparedness?

The FAO and World Bank have both reported the need for increased funds to effectively deal with the H5N1 virus in poultry. This does not imply that resources should be diverted from human preparedness, but that many of the most severely affected countries do not have adequate resources in veterinary medicine, agriculture, and research to develop and implement a successful eradication program from poultry in the near future. That is part of the reason that USDA and several federal agency partners are working with the international community to assist countries affected by H5N1 with prevention and response efforts.

Domestically the United States government is taking a proactive approach to ensure that there is a plan in place to combat both a human and an animal outbreak. USDA is working to ensure that we can detect, contain, isolate, and eradicate any outbreaks of H5N1.

Do you believe that H5N1 can be controlled in birds?

H5N1 HPAI (highly pathogenic avian influenza) virus has been effectively eradicated in three countries during 2004—Japan, South Korea, and Malaysia. They used time-tested plus new technologies as part of the effective eradication program. Other countries have not been as successful at elimination. This does not mean they cannot eliminate the virus from their country, but that new strategies need to be developed and implemented, including improving veterinary medical infrastructure and research to develop better diagnostic tools and improved strategies to protect birds from infection.

Here in the United States, we continue to work . . . to ensure we are prepared to respond to any HPAI outbreaks, including H5N1.

Do you believe that we are missing the forest by focusing on this one tree? Are we misinforming the public about H5N1 by not focusing on the issue of avian flu viruses in general?

There are 16 hemagglutinin and 9 neuraminidase subtypes of avian influenza viruses, for a potential of 144 different subtypes. Some of these subtypes have caused outbreaks in domestic poultry in the past. There are . . . 24 epizootics of the highly pathogenic avian influenza (HPAI) virus. . . . You can see the importance of other subtypes of the HPAI viruses. In addition, there are significant outbreaks of the H9N2 low pathogenicity avian influenza (LPAI) virus, which is endemic in poultry in much of Middle East and Asia. We are continually examining the subtypes that emerge and cause infection in poultry within different parts of the world.

Are there other avian flu viruses we should be more concerned about?

Other subtypes of AI virus have caused outbreaks in poultry and associated human infections. However, not all AI viruses have had the same risk to infect humans and should not be placed in the same category as the Asian H5N1 HPAI viruses. In several of the HPAI outbreaks, no evidence of human infection was detected, plus some experimental studies have shown not all HPAI viruses have a high risk for human infection (Dybing et al.). In summary, there is no evidence to suggest that there are currently other avian influenza viruses that we should be more concerned about, but we recognize that others have caused human illness and that any influenza virus has the potential to cause illness, thus our vigilant research and surveillance efforts.

What plan does the USDA have in mind for (1) preventing H5N1 from coming here and (2) controlling it if it does?

USDA is taking several steps to prevent the spread of H5N1 HPAI. Those efforts begin at the source, in countries affected by the virus. USDA is working with several of our federal partners to assist those countries with prevention and response efforts. USDA also maintains trade restrictions on the importation of poultry and poultry products from countries affected by H5N1. Furthermore, all imported live birds are quarantined and tested. The elaborate surveillance system in place in the United States is also important. USDA works with federal, state, and industry partners to monitor commercial flocks, live bird markets, backyard flocks, and migratory bird populations. In the event of an outbreak, USDA is prepared to work closely with state governments to quickly contain, isolate, and eradicate the disease.

Visitor to the land of the sneezing duck

A week before Thanksgiving, I received a worried phone call from my patient Mike Lee. It was the first I'd heard from him in more than two years. Before this call, Mike had always displayed a calm, easy manner.

"Bird flu is going to kill my business," he practically shouted over the phone, clearly much more afraid of a loss of income than any direct physical threat from the bird flu itself.

Mr. Lee had stopped coming to see me for his high blood pressure back in early 2003 when his Asia travel business was almost destroyed by SARS. He had lost his health insurance and was too depressed to tell me about it, although in other similar situations I would often see a patient free of charge.

Somehow he had hung on to the business. In 2005 he'd finally made it profitable again, but now he was being slammed by bird flu. SARS had faded, but the entire culture of Asia was connected to birds. Birds walked the streets; poultry were killed in open pits on farms. How was bird flu possibly going to be wiped out? Mr. Lee felt bad for the birds, but people were going to suffer tremendous financial hardship from fear of the birds. "How am I going to get through this virus?" he moaned on the phone, almost as if he had it.

He came to my office the next day and sat in my consultation room on the small blue leather couch across from me. He was usually a quiet man, but I could see he was in a mood to talk. He talked about the start of his now dying tour business. He had first traveled to Bangkok twenty years before while working as an engineer for a telecommunications company. Bangkok is still a study in the kind of contrasts that make the spread of bird flu possible. There is deeply entrenched poverty amid emerging wealth. There are brand-new Mercedes driving past people with tin roofs on their homes.

When I asked him about the safety of traveling to Asia over the years, he smiled for the first time. "Don't drink the tap water; fruits and vegetables should be peeled, rinsed, and preferably cooked."

"What about birds?"

Lee sighed. "In the small villages of Southeast Asia, chickens are everywhere. They also become like pets for many families. In the markets chickens are usually sold live. There are no supermarkets except in the largest cities. Bird sellers keep their birds in cages, sometimes several birds to a cage. And if a bird in the cage dies, it just sits there with the live ones. Cages of chickens are kept next to cages of ducks or even pigeons. At the end of the day the unsold birds go back home, even if they had shared a cage with a dead bird. The richer countries like Japan have better conditions."

He shook his head. "At home in Vietnam the kids may play with the chickens. Or the males may be taken to the local cockfights. The conditions for the birds are really bad. The bird owners use a lot of tricks to get their birds in fighting mood, and a popular way is to put the bird's beak in the owner's mouth, to wet the beak with saliva. It gets a bird really cranked."

"So it's not surprising," I said, "that several of the people who've gotten bird flu have lived in Vietnam."

Mike Lee has sent many different groups of people to Asia. Businesspeople go there for trade. Academics and students go for classes and teaching engagements and conferences. Tourists go to walk on China's Great Wall or cruise the rivers or visit the temples. Scientists, artists, backpackers, filmmakers, shoppers, and others travel to Asia to experience the culture. "But," Mr. Lee said, "none of them handle or kiss live birds."

Mr. Lee told me he believes that increased trade and tourism has helped to raise standards of living in most of Asia, and hopefully will help eliminate the breeding grounds for the new diseases of the future. Not long ago, he points out, it was usual to see "honeypots" (waste carriers) being transported on all the streets of Asia. But postwar development led to improved sanitary conditions, and honeypots are now disappearing even in the poorer countries. With increased wealth come healthier ways to grow and sell birds, as well as better access to health care.

"The Asian travel business employs millions of people," Mr. Lee said. "Some work in hotels or airports or restaurants or shops in Asia. Others bring outside business like I do. When their jobs are threatened or lost they lose their health. They get sick, but it's not from bird flu. It's starvation, hepatitis, or AIDS."

I spoke with Mike Lee about aiming his tour business at a different part of the world that wasn't being damaged by the latest health threat. I also treated his growing depression with a pill.

Lee said he wasn't ready to give up on Asia. He would try to ride out bird flu just as he had ridden out SARS. Modern technology was bringing better health to the birds and people of Asia, making them less of a health threat to us. Meanwhile, people like Lee continue to treasure the old while at the same time bringing in the new.

He told me wistfully about a Buddhist monastery in southeastern China, where tourists traveled to see a thousand-year-old kitchen with a fire that has been burning for over six hundred years.

I felt inadequate giving him a Prozac prescription as he was leaving. Here was the one patient who wasn't frantic years in advance of a bird disease that still barely affected humans, and yet he was the one I was treating for depression rather than the hysterical nontravelers who were costing him his job.

5

TAMIFLU AND THE BIRD FLU VACCINE

Back in 2001, when twenty-two people developed anthrax via spores sent through the mail, fear of the mail became so great that thirty thousand people took the antibiotic ciprofloxacin as a form of protection or preventative. In fact, this antibiotic can cause diarrhea, insomnia, and rashes, and neurological symptoms in children. But when people are afraid, they look for something to calm them, and the urge to combat the supposed danger unleashes a powerful emotion. The problem wasn't anthrax, it was fear of anthrax, and Cipro was a Band-Aid for that fear.

I remember one patient back in 2001 who became so contorted with anthrax fear that I barely recognized him, though he had been coming to see me for almost ten years. It wasn't that his appearance had changed, though the baseball cap pulled low over his eyes and the work-man's shoes were not his usual attire.

Under the lights of my examination room, I realized that it was his manner that had altered the most. For-merly confident, even strident, he now leaned against the counter, not wanting to sit. He hunched over, wring-ing his hands, looking every few seconds toward the window.

Seeing me, he seemed to calm, and I reminded him that the visit was a simple follow-up for a prostate infection. He needed to leave a urine sample and he could go, and I would call him in a few days with the results. He could stop taking his Cipro.

"I've renewed it," he whispered, though his voice usu-ally boomed.

"Why renew it? I gave you the refill in case the infec-tion flared up again and you couldn't reach me right away."

"Why should I stop now?" And then came the words that were supposed to explain everything: "There's a war on."

I could see him eyeing the closets in the examination room. Was he wondering what medicines were there? I put my hand on his shoulder, and we looked at each other. I realized that I had always treated this patient more like a friend. He knew my home phone number; he was free to page me when I wasn't on call. We liked to talk about sports. It was painful to consider a new out-side tension that had become the order of the day between us.

In my consultation room I explained to the patient that the risks of taking this expensive antibiotic for an extended period far outweighed any benefit against an inconceivable microbe. With prolonged use of the medicine this patient might develop diarrhea, rash, or insomnia.

"Insomnia," he said. "So what? I already can't sleep."

I reviewed my office notes and noted that a few years before he'd had a brief spell of anxiety related to a problem at work. He had declined medication, and the problem had resolved on its own.

"How about something to calm your nerves and help you sleep?"

The patient readily agreed this time. He was thirty-five, lived alone in a walk-up apartment six blocks from the World Trade Center site. He worked uptown at a communications firm and had been at work when the planes hit, but soon after he had returned to a smoky, soot-covered existence downtown, where he had to keep the windows closed and his telephone hadn't worked for weeks. He told me that since September 11 he spent the night sitting in a chair, fully clothed, in case he had to leave at a moment's notice.

I tried my best to reassure him. "Nothing else is likely to happen right now. The risk of anthrax is extraordinarily low. Don't you believe me?"

"Sure I believe you, Doc. But I just can't stop thinking about it."

Across my desk I could see his bulky bag, bulging open with a gas mask. He said he carried it wherever he went. I tried not to look at it. "Would you agree to see a therapist?"

"Are you saying I'm crazy?"

"Of course not. I'm worried that your reaction is causing you pain."

"I can handle it. Let's talk about something more important. The vaccine for anthrax? Can you get it?"

"It's not a very strong vaccine, and you can't get it here in America right now. If you insist on it, you can fly to England to get it."

"Are you crazy, Doc? Me get on a plane right now?"

The patient rose and headed to the front of the office. I felt that my "plane" suggestion had caused him to lose some respect for me.

"Wait," I said. But he ignored me. He was heading for my supply closet at the front of the office. Without hesitation, he began rummaging through it.

My nurse, who had never before seen a patient so boldly enter a private area of the office, seemed afraid to intervene. The patient knocked over pillboxes until he found the antibiotic he was looking for, and then he stuffed it into his pockets until my supply was exhausted. He left the office then, without saying good-bye to anyone.

I found myself ready to enter the hall after him, but my nurse wisely stopped me. "Let him go," she said.

Tamiflu is the new Cipro

In 2005, the Cipro man was still coming to see me. He had long since discarded his Cipro, and he no longer slept with his boots on. Still he worried. When the bird flu scare hit, he was one of the first to ask if he could have a supply of Tamiflu on hand just in case. I told him that Tamiflu was unproven against bird flu in humans, and that since there weren't even any cases here in birds, we would all be better off if we left decisions about emergency stockpiles to the government.

"The government," he snorted. "What do they know."

All the same, I told the patient I didn't believe in personal stockpiles, period. I felt a physician had an intrinsic role in deciding if and when a medication was prescribed. Tamiflu seemed to be a relatively safe drug. It had been given to 32 million people since its inception in 1999, with the most common side effect being nausea (5 to 10 percent). Recently, in Japan, where 24 million prescriptions had been written, the Japanese Health Ministry revealed that thirty-two people were noted to have psychiatric problems and twelve people had died, though an FDA panel here in the United States reported that no cause and effect had been shown. It was clear that Tamiflu needed further study, but for the moment it was still considered quite safe.

"Is Tamiflu safe?" he asked me.

My patient said he knew about these Japanese reports, and he was afraid the drug would make him anxious. He'd always admitted to me that he was an anxious patient, though he probably thought he was less anxious than he actually was. Perhaps this was why he didn't press me for it—his fear of bird flu was being temporarily overcome by his fear of Tamiflu. In any case, I didn't have any samples of the drug in my closet, so his willpower couldn't be tested as it had been back in 2001.

If the worst-case scenario occurred and there was a new pandemic, I suspected that Tamiflu might be useful. How useful it would be depended on how extensive the pandemic. The last two pandemics in 1957 and 1968 had been relatively mild, and the swine flu scare in 1976 had been about fear rather than flu. Of the four anti-flu drugs on the market in 2005, Tamiflu was the newest, seemingly the best tolerated, and the one that had been shown to work as a preventative. But preventative against what? The 32 million previous users had taken Tamiflu to ward off or treat human influenza, which claimed thirty-six thousand lives in the United States every year. Tamiflu lessened symptoms and duration by at least one day. But for bird flu? Since there was currently no bird flu in the United States, the Tamiflu stockpiles were a treatment for fear rather than bird flu. There was no justifying any potential side effects when there was no disease to treat.

Many patients were misinformed that Tamiflu was some kind of vaccine, rather than a drug that reduced symptoms by blocking viral spread within an infected host. But my Cipro patient knew exactly what Tamiflu was. He must have decided he would overcome his fear of the Japanese side effects, because he asked me for some samples "just in case."

"They don't bring us samples of Tamiflu," I replied.

Now he didn't know what to do. He began to clench and unclench his fists. He needed an instant treatment against the fear of bird flu. I knew without asking that he wasn't eating chicken, had long ago removed the bird feeder from his backyard, and carefully avoided pigeon droppings on the street.

But none of that was enough. This patient needed a vaccine against the fear of bird flu. Since the bird flu vaccine itself wasn't yet available for that purpose, he asked me for the next best thing, the yearly flu vaccine.

In fact, in 2005 the obsession with bird flu had taken attention away from the yearly flu shot, which the year before had appeared like a panacea in the face of a sudden shortage. When a prop against fear is lacking, the threat itself always seems more ominous.

But in 2005, the year's regular flu was forgotten, overcome by the sinister threat of those monstrously ill Asian birds.

All at once my patient said excitedly, "Hey, do you have any flu vaccine in yet?"

I answered in the affirmative. I'd just received my yearly supply a few days before. I could see what he was thinking—the yearly flu vaccine must also offer him some protection against bird flu.

I vaccinated him, treating his fear, but I didn't have the heart to tell him that there was simply no evidence that it would arm his immune system against the H5N1 bird flu virus.

What is Tamiflu?

There are four anti-flu drugs currently on the market, amantadine, rimantadine, Relenza, and Tamiflu. All four drugs have been shown to reduce the duration of flu symptoms by one day if taken within the first two days of the onset of the flu.

Amantadine has been on the market since 1976. Rimantadine, which works in the same way, was added in 1993. These drugs work by interfering with the virus's ability to make copies of itself. Though there are many strains of influenza, they all have the same viral protein, M2, and amantadine and rimantadine are effective against strains of influenza A (including H5N1). However, a recent study in a British journal revealed a developing drug resistance—meaning the virus strain had become resistant, not the patient—in 12 percent of cases. It may soon become useless in avian viruses as well, as China has apparently been administering billions of doses of amantadine to poultry (something banned in most of the West). This growing drug resistance is part of what has led to the development of new drugs that work in a different way.

Relenza and Tamiflu appeared in 1999 and are effective against both influenza A and B. Relenza is an inhaleable powder, so it has limited use in asthmatics and others with respiratory difficulties. These two drugs are called neuraminidase inhibitors, which means that they block the enzymes that dot the surface of flu viruses. (Neuraminidase is the N1 in H5N1.) As I've mentioned previously, neuraminidase enzymes help to make and then break the bonds that hold a flu virus to the outside of cells and thereby help it spread to other cells in the host. Neuraminidase inhibitors prevent the viral spread.

All four anti-flu drugs are similarly effective and are approved for use in children older than one year, but amantadine and rimantadine can cause nervousness, anxiety, insomnia, difficulty concentrating, and light-headedness (13 percent in amantadine, 6 percent in rimantadine). Nausea occurs in about 2 percent of patients taking amantadine or rimantadine, and at least three times as often in patients taking Tamifu.

Only Tamiflu has been studied as a preventative against the flu (rather than simply a treatment for it), and it is that designation that makes it the ready drug to stockpile against bird flu. In fact, it has only been studied—and found to be moderately effective—against the H5N1 virus in mice, though it is anticipated to have some effect in humans even if the H5N1 virus mutates.

But part of the difficulty with stockpiling this drug is the lack of a clear indication of when to take it. If a bird in the United States gets bird flu? Definitely not. If a bird in your neighborhood is infected? Here, too, there would be no indication, since it is almost impossible to contract bird flu from casual contact with a bird.

Even if the worst-case scenario occurs and the current deadly bird flu virus mutates into a form that is still lethal and passes human to human, and even if Tamiflu maintains its effectiveness against the mutated virus, it still wouldn't be clear when to take it. When the mutated bug enters the country? When it is found in your neighborhood? Certainly one would consider taking it if someone in the family contracted the dread disease, a prospect that is currently quite remote.

Voyeuristic attachment to cable news reports makes the bird flu appear to be too looming, too imminent, too much of a personal threat. This leads to a stockpiling of Tamiflu, a drug with side effects (most commonly nausea, but with the remote possibility of neurological or psychiatric symptoms). Tamiflu is a drug, like its three cousins, that was intended to lessen the symptoms of an ongoing bout of the flu. It certainly makes sense to consider it if that flu is a more powerful pandemic strain, whether it initiates from the deadly H5N1 bird flu virus or not. But Tamiflu is not a vaccine, and it does not make sense for people to stockpile it now for expected prophylactic use in the immediate future. Not only will those stockpiles cost money, but they will also expire in about three years.

The bird flu vaccine

Vaccine-making resources in the United States are stretched thin. There are just three manufacturers responsible for making more than 80 million doses of the yearly human flu vaccine, with no guarantee that the entire supply will be sold or adequately distributed. The Food and Drug Administration tries to ensure that the vaccine supply is sterile, an expensive proposition for a drug manufacturer, especially when dealing with a generic product such as a vaccine. In 2004, the entire 50-million-dose batch that Chiron (a U.S. company whose manufacturing plant is in Great Britain) made had to be discarded because it was found to be contaminated with a common bacteria known as serratia.

As recently as the 1970s, there were twenty-seven vaccine makers in the United States. But because of the narrow profit margin and fear of litigation, many manufacturers left the game. Fearful of a pandemic, Tommy Thompson, the former secretary of the U.S. Department of Health and Human Services, beginning in 2002 requested at least $100 million three years in row to upgrade the country's vaccine capability. The money was to be used to help the vaccine industry switch over from using chicken eggs to make vaccines to a new cell-based technology using genetic technology.

The first year, Congress cut all of his request. The second year, he got half of what he asked for. Finally, in 2004, after a public outcry over a flu vaccine shortage that year, the entire $100 million was approved.

But even at a time of such great difficulty with the flu vaccine supply, the post-9/11 era, the vaccine focus in Congress has been elsewhere. In early 2005, a powerful group of Republican lawmakers began pushing "BioShield 2" through Congress. The original BioShield, signed into law in July 2004, allocated $5.6 billion dollars over ten years to the Department of Homeland Security for the purchase of countermeasures against anthrax, smallpox, and other terrorist threats. This expenditure includes allocation for 75 million doses of a second-generation anthrax vaccine to be made available for stockpiling.

BioShield 2 proposes to shield the drug companies against lawsuits, one of their major disincentives against making vaccines, while expanding by several more billions the money allocated.

The federal government's vaccine focus switched dramatically to bird flu in the fall of 2005, when articles in *Nature* and *Science* disclosed the final sequencing of the 1918 Spanish flu H1N1 molecules. The fact that the Spanish flu was a bird flu had been known for at least thirty years, and the exact way it made its jump to humans was known for at least a year. Nevertheless, these studies, combined with the continued spread of H5N1 among the birds of Asia and on to Europe, fueled a public worry that was useful to public health officials who wanted more attention put on avian flu in general and on the bird flu vaccine in particular.

A vaccine against H5N1 had already been developed using a virus isolated from a Vietnamese patient in 2004. In late 2005, the National Institute was testing this vaccine against humans, and according to Dr. Anthony Fauci, director of the National Institute of Allergy and Infectious Diseases (NAID), it had been shown to be safe and to induce an immune response that is predictive of being protective. Fauci also has indicated in the media that there is currently not enough vaccine production capacity to make enough for people who might need it.

Of course, Fauci was referring again to the worst-case scenario: if a mutation occurred to allow the H5N1 virus to pass from human to human, and if this virus maintained its lethality (as I pointed out in chapter 4, it is actually difficult to determine how lethal it is), and if it spreads here and becomes a pandemic among humans. Both the CDC and the NIH have indicated that the goal would be to produce 300 million doses in six months if it appeared that the worst-case scenario was imminent. The current Health and Human Services secretary, Mike Leavitt, has said that it would take three to five years under the current system to reach the point where such rapid production is possible. (In 1976, the rapid turn-around of vaccine was more easily accomplished because the climate of vaccine production was better. In fact, it was partly the swine flu fiasco that scared vaccine manu-facturers away.)

Leavitt advocates a stepped-up government involve-ment in the production of flu vaccines both for a possible pandemic as well as for the yearly vaccine. He believes in using federal statutes to limit the liability of the drug companies while providing compensation for those who are inadvertently hurt by a vaccine. He believes in involving the FDA in the process so that there is regula-tory flexibility, while guaranteeing a market to the drug companies for the vaccines that are ultimately developed.

The *Milwaukee Journal Sentinel*, in an article entitled "Are We Prepared?" on November 13, 2005, indicated that the Department of Health and Human Services had come up with a list of who would get the vaccine first. These two groups (health care workers and vaccine mak-ers) would require 10 million doses. Next would come people with chronic illnesses, the immuno-compromised, and those over sixty-five. Unfortunately, by publicly focusing on this list, as well as the attempts to upgrade vaccine-making capabilities to the point where the entire population could be covered, the government once again sent the unintended message that a large pandemic was in the offing, though in fact it remained a low-probability event.

Three to five years?

How could it take three to five years to get a vaccine ready that would be needed in just months in order to save lives? Could our system really be that out of date?

At the end of October 2005, President Bush had proposed to Congress a $7.1 billion expenditure to deal with the avian flu risk. Happily, this plan included $2.7 billion to upgrade vaccine manufacture using the modern cell-based technology and a strategy to decrease the liability to vaccine manufacturers so they would be inclined to participate.

After clueless unprepared hospitals, the second-weakest link in our preparation chain is vaccine production. When we vaccinate, a dead or weakened virus is injected into a person, where it generates an immune response, but without causing any symptoms of the disease it is meant to protect you from. The body then carries, for some extended period of time, the specific antibodies for that virus or bacteria and has the capacity to make more if actually challenged by that virus or bacteria.

Though genetic recombinant techniques are routinely used for other vaccines such as hepatitis (an E. coli bacteria is "programmed" to make viral antibody), and have been since the 1980s, the United States still currently produces all influenza vaccines, including potential bird flu vaccines, using a method created almost fifty years ago. First, scientists identify the live virus from the blood of a victim. Next, it is injected into a fertilized chicken egg.

Once it's been grown in chicken eggs, it has to be injected into more chicken eggs, until millions of eggs have been injected with the virus. The virus is harvested, purified, and then neutralized. It may take half a year or more from finding the strain to releasing the first set of vaccine doses to the public.

Ironically, the H5N1 virus is so deadly to chicken embryos that it interferes with the process to make a vaccine against itself. The eggs have to be specially treated so they can be used.

The technology is available but expensive to change over to state-of-the-art methods. The most commonly used methods involve reverse genetics and cell cultures.

In reverse genetics, you don't need the original strain of the virus to work from. Using the structure of the virus, scientists can genetically engineer an influenza virus they already have to present a different H and a different N, inserting strips of genetic material, turning one viral strain into another. Then, instead of injecting that genetically manipulated strain into a million eggs, they grow it with cell cultures.

First, scientists grow animal cells or human cells in big vats of a nutrient solution. Then they inject the virus strain, created via reverse genetics, into the cells. As the cells reproduce, so does the virus. Eventually the outer wall of cell is removed, and the viruses are harvested, purified, and then neutralized or killed. Once dead, they can safely be injected into subjects as a vaccine, inducing an animal or a person to make antibodies against this "manufactured" virus. Using this method, the interval between identifying a strain and producing the first batch of vaccines can be measured in days instead of months.

BIRD FLU

So why do we still rely on the chicken eggs? The answer is that vaccine manufacturers, although they use these techniques routinely for other viruses, have been reluctant to switch with flu vaccines because of expense as well as potential liability. Simply put, they don't know what side effects will occur until they start to test people. But the time to test a new vaccine is not in the middle of a pandemic. The time is now.

More research needs to be done to rule out the possibility of side effects. And after that, the Food and Drug Administration would have to approve it for human use—something it has yet to do.

On the horizon are other exciting advanced techniques, including one that targets the M2 protein of the influenza molecule. Since that molecule doesn't change, this kind of vaccine might provide immunity to all flus (including bird flu) for a decade rather than to one flu for one year only.

Molecular virologist Mittal Suresh and collaborators at Purdue University in Indiana are working on an adenovirus vector with funding from NIAID. This virus won't cause disease but can be injected with bird flu components and hopefully provide immunity.

And then there's Jose Galarza. In a tiny lab perched above the Hudson River, Galarza has been experimenting with tiny specks of genetic matter for nearly ten years. He works with microscopic blobs of genes (called viral-like particles, or VLPs), from which he fashions painless, oral vaccines more rapidly than traditional methods. In fact, Galarza believes he can command his VLPs to knock out bird flu in lab animals—and potentially in humans— more quickly and safely than conventional vaccines.

At the same time Bush announced the stockpiling and

102

money for new research, a similar vaccine was being used to inoculate millions of birds in Southeast Asia. This vaccine was able to be rushed into production because the same level of sterility and predictability necessary for humans doesn't apply to drugs for animals. The vaccine is useful in birds to immunize possible bird contacts of infected birds, but has its limitations.

Culling birds is still a more effective strategy to eradicate the disease. The vaccine is useful in target bird populations, but it is not powerful enough to bring about immunity in all cases. Partial immunity could convert potential victims (birds that would die and therefore not be able to spread the disease) into hosts that would survive and spread the virus.

In humans, an overall immunization strategy makes more sense, since the goal is to decrease the death rate and the severity of the illness. If a worst-case scenario were to occur, we would need a modern vaccine to be able to combat it.

Part II

THE EVOLUTION OF BIRD FLU CONCERNS

6

OUR CULTURE OF FEAR

Can we cure fear?

In early 2004 my daughter, Rebecca, was taking a bath. She was almost three years old, the time when the brain circuitry completes its wiring of the "safety center" in the prefrontal cortex. When the tub's Jacuzzi device turned on, she became petrified. I raced to her side, to find her standing straight up, bright red from crying.

For months afterward, she abhorred baths. As a physician who has studied fear, I tried to appeal to her newly working brain center to suppress the worry that this tub would always bring the scary bubbles, but her body's innate response was too strong. By starting with showers and diverting the focus of her attention from the tub, I was gradually able to return her to baths. But to this day she is wary of bubbles.

Why is fear so intractable? And what can we do about it? Therapy has provided succor for many people; others have relied on the strength they get from their faiths or other support networks. But—in a world where we are regularly exposed to hair-raising events such as the full-color aftermath of suicide bomber attacks beamed into our living room TVs as well as the ominous forecasts of the next pandemic—is such verbal support enough? Answering that need, fear-blunting medications are coming onto the scene. Could we—should we all—simply pop pills to ease our anxieties?

The roots of fear

Fear is more than a state of mind; it is chemical. The feeling of alarm arises from the circuitry of our brains, in the neurochemical exchanges between nerve cells. Fear is a physical reaction to a perceived threat. As long as the danger is direct and real, fear is normal and helps protect us. Fear also has a genetic component. A rat will respond to the odor of a fox, even if that rodent has spent its whole life in a laboratory. Likewise, we humans are automatically apprehensive about situations that threatened our ancestors.

When an individual feels threatened, the metabolism revs up in anticipation of an imminent need to defend oneself or flee. "Fight or flight," or the acute stress response, was first described by Walter Cannon, an American physiologist, in the 1920s. Cannon observed that animals, including humans, react to dangers with a hormonal discharge of the nervous system. The body unleashes an outpouring of vessel-constricting, heart-thumping hormones, including epinephrine, norepinephrine, and the steroid cortisol. The heart speeds up and pumps harder, the nerves fire more quickly, the skin cools and gets goose bumps, the eyes dilate to see better, and the areas of the brain involved in initiating action receive a message that it is time to do something.

At the center of these processes is the amygdala, an almond-shaped region of the brain. Neuroscientist Joseph E. LeDoux of New York University, a pioneer in the study of the fear cycle, describes the amygdala as "the hub in the brain's wheel of fear." The amygdala processes the primitive emotions of fear, hate, love, bravery, and anger—all neighbors in the deep limbic brain we inherit from animals that developed earlier. The amygdala works together with other brain centers that feed it or respond to it. This fear hub senses through the thalamus (the brain's receiver), analyzes with the cortex (the brain's seat of reasoning), and remembers via the hippocampus (the brain's file cabinet).

It takes only 12 milliseconds, according to LeDoux, for the thalamus to process sensory input and signal the amygdala. He calls this emotional brain the "low road." The high road, or the thinking brain, takes 30 to 40 milliseconds to process what is happening. The hippo-campal memory center provides the context. "People have fear they don't understand or can't control because it is processed by the low road," LeDoux says.

The fear factor

Once a person has learned to fear something, he may always feel dread associated with that experience. But unlike mice, we humans can also be alarmed by events we have only read or heard about, so we may worry about disasters we may never experience. If we are unable to respond for lack of an appropriate target, the fear accumulates and we become anxious.

This cycle can become self-perpetuating. My eight-year-old son, Joshua, for example, has been afraid of dogs since he was terrified at the age of two by a sudden barking he heard when we were hiking on a mountain trail. I said, "The dog is gone," but he said, "No, it's not. It keeps coming back."

Now each time a dog barks, it engages the same mechanism. My son's thalamus triggers his amygdala, which retrieves the fearful memory for him from the hippocampus, and his body goes into hyperdrive. This is a warning system malfunction, because it is alerting him to a danger that doesn't actually threaten him.

In studies of how humans evaluate risks, psychologists Robert J. and Caroline Blanchard at the University of Hawaii at Manoa have found that people often fail to assess the level of threat accurately. We tend to over-personalize risk and to experience an unrealistic sense of danger whenever we hear or read of a bad event occurring to someone else.

For example, my mother-in-law has a severe case of multiple sclerosis and has been confined to a wheelchair for almost twenty years. Six years ago, my brother-in-law developed a mild case of MS, and my wife, a neurologist, then confided in me her fear, practically a conviction, that she would be next. Every time she brings up her perception that MS is her destiny, I try to counter it with the bald statistic that only 4 percent of close relatives are at risk for the disease. "There is a 96 percent chance that you won't get it," I say. But for my wife, as for many others, the perception rests with the 4 percent.

Empathy for her mother and a natural tendency to personalize her experience create the fear and the conviction, despite her neurologist's knowledge of the disease.

Recurrent or unremitting fear has the same deleterious effects on the human body that running persistently at 80 to 100 mph has on a car. Many illnesses are more likely to occur as a result, including heart disease, stroke, and depression. What we have most to be concerned about are not the extraordinary occurrences or exotic diseases, however, but the ordinary killers such as heart attacks that develop as a result of our incessant worries. Consider: in 2001 terrorists killed 2,978 people in the United States, including the 5 from anthrax. That same year, according to the Centers for Disease Control, heart disease killed 700,142; cancer, 553,768; accidents, 101,537; and suicide, 30,622. Murders (not including 9/11) accounted for 17,330 deaths.

The wrong worries

At a time in history when true scourges are quite rare, the population is controlled by fear. Rather than enjoy the safety that our technological advances have provided us, we feel uncertain. Respiratory masks and other paraphernalia meant to shield us actually spread panic more effectively than any terrorist agent by sending the message that something is in the offing. Our personal fear alerts are turned on all the time.

We feel the stress and become more prone to irritability, disagreement, worry, insomnia, anxiety, and depression. We are more likely to experience chest pain, shortness of breath, dizziness, and headache. We become more prone to heart disease, cancer, and stroke, our greatest killers. Worry about the wrong things puts us at greater risk of the diseases that should be concerning us in the first place.

The connection between excess worry and increased disease risk is not just hypothetical. Numerous studies have shown a link between stress reported by patients and ill health. Special health conditions for which research has shown an impact from stress include:

- *Heart disease, cancer, chronic lung disease* A study in the *American Journal of Preventive Medicine* (1998) shows a strong relationship between childhood anxiety, growing out of a dysfunctional household, and multiple risk factors for leading causes of death in adults including heart disease, cancer, and lung disease.

- *Coronary heart disease* The American Heart Association cites research linking stress, socioeconomic status, and health behaviors with coronary heart disease risk. Stress may affect behavior. For example, people under stress may overeat, start smoking, or smoke more than they otherwise would.

- *Cancer* Some studies of women with breast cancer have shown significantly higher rates of disease among women who experienced traumatic life events and losses within several years before diagnosis. Although studies have shown that stress factors (such as death of a spouse, social isolation, and medical school examinations) alter the way the immune system functions, they have not provided scientific evidence of a direct cause-and-effect relationship between these immune system changes and the development of cancer. Many factors come into play when determining the relationship between stress and cancer. At present, the relationship between psychological stress and cancer occurrence or progression has not been scientifically proven.

- *Stroke*   A study of more than two thousand middle-aged men between ages forty-nine and sixty-four, in the journal *Stroke* (2002), showed three times greater incidence of fatal stroke for those suffering from depression or anxiety.

- *Wound healing*   An Australian study published in December 2005 shows that an increased neuro-peptide level during stress disrupts wound healing. Another study from Ohio State released at the same time reveals that marital strife diminishes the ability to heal physical wounds.

- *Overall health*   Studies in Israel have shown a cumulative effect of terrorism and fear on health. Suicide bombings in 2001 were shown to impact the personal sense of safety in 2002. A study that appeared in July 2004 in the journal *Psychosomatic Medicine* showed twice as high a level of an enzyme that correlates with heart disease among Israeli women who expressed fear of terrorism than among similar women who weren't worried.

Our culture of fear

In recent years the climate of fear has changed. Statistically, the industrialized world has never been safer. Many of us are living longer and more uneventfully. Nevertheless, we live in fear of worst-case scenarios. Over the past century, armed with scientific and technological breakthroughs, we Americans have dramatically reduced our risk in virtually every area of life, resulting in life spans 60 percent longer in 2000 than in 1900. Antibiotics have reduced the likelihood of dying from infections. It used to be that a person could die from a scratch. Now we gobble down antibiotics at the first sign of trouble. Public health measures dictate standards for drinkable water and breathable air. Our garbage is removed quickly. We live temperature-controlled, disease-controlled lives.

And yet, we worry more than ever before. The natural dangers are no longer there, but the response mechanisms are still in place, and now they are turned on much of the time. We implode, turning our adaptive fear mechanism into a maladaptive panicked response.

We are bombarded with information. We live by TV sound bite and by Internet hyperbite. Medical information has become agenda-driven, exaggerated by the media and disseminated on the Internet. The expectation of perfect health is perpetuated by these sources. Illness is no longer accepted as part of the natural order of things, and as consumers, we have become terrified of all disease, even though most of the time, doctors can diagnose an illness and offer either a cure or an effective treatment. Still, we continue to worry.

Our brains are not being infiltrated or provoked to panic by accident. Since 9/11 especially, the government has exploited its role as our official protector, from Homeland Security to the Centers for Disease Control (CDC). Airport screeners and the FBI are supposedly the last line of defense between Osama bin Laden and the citizens of western Ohio. Every warning about a scary new disease, every report of terrorist chatter, and every ultra-frail senior citizen becomes a justification for some government worker's job, from a research scientist all the way to President Bush himself. Government officials and politicians employ the media megaphone to promote the idea that they are keeping the populace safe. Unfortunately, there is no evidence that ongoing terror alerts correlate with the actual risk of a potential attack.

After a while the public becomes desensitized and can't tell a real alert from the latest hype. For example, promoting worst-case scenarios with biological or chemical weapons that may easily be blown away by the wind or destroyed by heat is a form of propaganda that makes people afraid and ready to comply with the government's agenda. It is misleading to call nerve gas or anthrax weapons of mass destruction when these are more likely tools that terrorists would use on a smaller scale. It would be extremely difficult to deploy chemical or biological agents to large numbers of potential victims at once. Drone planes seeding the air would likely be shot down before they could complete their tasks.

Of course, government officials can't grab the media megaphone if the media themselves don't make it available. The mass media tend to magnify the latest health concern and broadcast it to millions of people at once. This has the effect of elevating an issue to a grand scale and provoking panic way out of proportion to the risks. I call this phenomenon the "bug du jour." The craze of the moment appears to be a threat to our personal safety until it runs its course through the media spotlight. And when a new threat hits, private companies take their cues from media outlets and begin to line up for profit.

Why have we become so defenseless?

When Lyme disease, a troublesome bacteria transmitted to humans by the bite of a deer tick, was being hyped ten years ago, one of my most rational patients, a mathematics professor, was certain he had it every time he got a rash, even when he was living in Los Angeles, a city with zero deer.

"The chances of your having it are almost nonexistent," I assured him.

"Forget probabilities, I can just feel it," he said on more than one occasion.

Ten years later, with Lyme very much on the increase but out of the media spotlight, this patient—who by this time had moved to deer-ridden Connecticut—no longer had concerns about the now prevalent Lyme disease but worried instead about bioterrorism. As well as he understood probabilities and equations, when he turned on the news at night or read his newspaper in the morning, he often personalized the latest risk and became worried that he might die.

Like my professor patient, we absorb the sense of urgency and believe we are in danger. So busy are we with fake threats that we ignore real threats. With over 8 million cases of tuberculosis every year in the world, 5 million new cases of AIDS, over 300 million cases of malaria, and over a million deaths due to each, Americans rarely worry about these diseases. In the United States approximately 40,000 people die of influenza every year, a statistic that went unnoticed until 2003, when it was the flu's turn on the wheel of hype. In 2000, 63,000 Americans died of pneumonia, and 15,000 died of AIDS. This information stayed out of the news. In comparison to our real killer bugs, only 284 people died here of West Nile virus in 2002, when it was publicized by the media and perceived as a great threat.

In 2003, when Severe Acute Respiratory Syndrome (SARS) arrived and became almost synonymous with the word "virus," there were only 7,000 cases in the world, and fewer than 100 in the United States. No one here died of SARS, but a lot of people worried unnecessarily. Many patients called me in the spring of 2003 convinced that the slightest cough was SARS. People were afraid to sit next to an Asian person or to eat in a Chinese restaurant. Our public health system, specifically the World Health Organization and the CDC here in the United States, drove the media response to help contain SARS, quarantining Canada and most of Asia, and ultimately taking credit when SARS died down. Actually, there was no direct evidence that the massive travel alerts really squashed SARS as much as historically proven factors like isolating those who had the disease, as well as the arrival of summer, traditionally a difficult time for respiratory viruses to thrive. Still, the public perception was that SARS had gone overnight from being a worldwide threat in the spring of 2003 to being no threat at all by June. We braced ourselves for the next bug du jour and forgot all about SARS.

In the summer of 2003, we experienced a temporary reprieve—West Nile did not reappear on our media screens that summer, and hardly anyone was afraid that his next mosquito bite would be his last.

Many of the bugs du jour are cause for concern only among a narrow segment of the population. Only a small portion of those who believe they are at risk really are, and few who become infected actually die. But a strange disease that kills only a few people still makes for good headlines if the story is strategically hyped. Many news teasers use the line "Are you and your family at risk?"

The answer is usually no, but that tagline generates concern in every viewer, and this is what keeps people tuned in. If we didn't fundamentally misunderstand the risk, we probably wouldn't watch.

Each terror alert is like another bug du jour. We talk of sarin, which killed only twelve people in a Japanese subway in 1995 but panicked thousands, and can panic us here without so much as a single case. Anthrax infected twenty-two people through the U.S. mail in the fall of 2001, killing five unfortunate people, yet had thirty thousand more taking the antibiotic Cipro, many indiscriminately and without a doctor's prescription. It's hard to believe that there hasn't been a case of smallpox here since the 1940s, considering all the attention it has received. If it is ever again introduced into the population, it is likely to spread slowly, by respiratory droplet.

Meanwhile, in 2002, the fear of smallpox spread far more virulently through the public, transmitted by word of mouth. In the fall of 2004, the sudden shortage of flu vaccine in the United States led to a stampede of people seeking the coveted elixir. During this vaccine shortage, multitudes of healthy people became convinced that they could be overcome with the flu and die at any time. In fact, the first flu-related death that year came not from the disease, but from an elderly woman who fell while waiting for the vaccine amidst a thronging crowd. I wrote an op-ed piece in the *New York Post* pointing out that the CDC had determined that the vaccine hadn't helped much the year before, was only 40 to 60 percent effective, and was intended mostly for high-risk groups. My message:

flu vaccine is not the health panacea that you think it is, you are not in great danger without it, and the sudden attention it is receiving has caused people to feel a sense of urgency out of proportion to the real danger.

I thought I'd accomplished something until I began to receive phone calls from patients who had read my piece. Almost as an afterthought I'd mentioned that I had five vials, or fifty doses, to give to my sickest patients.

"I saw your article," one call began.

"Are you reassured?" I asked.

The patient ignored me. "I understand you have some vaccine. Can I have a shot?"

Rather than worrying less after learning the facts, each patient wanted to be one of the lucky fifty and was calling me to beg for a dose.

Reeducating the public when it came to panic was going to take far more than a corrective article that unintentionally became part of the hype. The year before, the deaths of a few children from flu in Colorado had led instantly to a nationwide panic before dropping from the news radar. Yet both years, despite all the concern, would turn out to be nonepidemic flu years.

When the media or the government focuses on the bug du jour, we all feel it, as though it's a palpable danger. When media attention is diverted elsewhere, the manifested fear fades but remains below the surface, waiting to attach itself to the next hyped target. At a time in history when there are no true scourges, the population is controlled through fear. Instead of enjoying the safety that our technological advances have provided us, we feel uncertain. Our personal fear alerts are constantly turned on. Fear is not intrinsically pathological; it is a reaction to the pathology of our times. Stress makes us more prone to irritability, anxiety, and depression, and we're more likely to experience physical symptoms such as chest pain, shortness of breath, dizziness, and headaches.

After weeks go by without our being shot by a sniper, bitten by a West Nile mosquito, gassed with sarin, or infected with SARS, people become desensitized. Each new phase of hysteria is followed by a brief period when our guard comes down.

But who can a frightened person count on for reliable information and reassurance?

Teachers absorb the same information fragments that students do, reinforcing the students' sense of fear. Patients fear becoming ill, they fear the onset of suffering, and yet, doctors specialize in, and are trained to treat, specific diseases rather than the patient as a whole.

Patients hover nervously around the medical secretary's desk as their diagnoses roll in via faxed reports. The pills are better, the surgeries are better, and the rehab techniques are better, but these positive developments are not enough to offset the fear of test results.

Expecting a problem-free life

Dr. Rachel Yehuda, an expert on posttraumatic stress, said she thinks we struggle as a society today because we feel entitled to live a trauma-free life. We ask, "Why me?" whereas "in a previous generation, no one had the expectation that something wouldn't happen to them—in those days, it was 'Why not me?' Previously, no one thought that being exposed to a trauma was that unusual.

"Posttraumatic stress is a mismatch between what we think the world should be like, and what it is really like.

We aren't prepared. In a culture where you're expecting people to hate you, you let go of it for a lot longer. In Europe, for example, Jews always had the thought that a certain percentage wouldn't survive because of anti-Semitism. There was a lower expectation of peaceful existence, so the trauma of threat was less."

Dr. Yehuda also indicated that many of our scientists and those who inform us do us a disservice by overdramatizing their concerns. This grandiosity is part of what causes the public to overperceive risks. "We scientists can't tolerate being cogs in a wheel. Technology allows us to look at things we never could before. But we need to learn to be excited by what we do without telling a premature story. We can alarm people unnecessarily. And then we're stuck with our story, right or wrong."

Assessing risk

We need to learn how to see risk in perspective, without overreacting to imagined dangers. Unfortunately, there is no consensus about what constitutes proper risk assessment or the best way to accomplish it. There is disagreement about who is an expert on risk, and some authors don't trust so-called experts at all because of their hidden agendas.

Published in 2002, David Ropeik and George Gray's book *Risk* is a practical guide intended to counter the hysteria caused by inaccurate public health reporting. These authors believe that "we live in a dangerous world. Yet it is also a world far safer in many ways than it has ever been. Life expectancy is up. Infant mortality is down. Diseases that only recently were mass killers have been all but eradicated. Advances in public health, medicine, environmental regulation, food safety, and worker protection have dramatically reduced many of the major risks we faced just a few decades ago."

Ropeik and Gray developed a risk meter, a way of converting uncertainty into calculable risk. This risk meter assesses the likelihood of exposure to a potential danger as well as the consequences if you are one of the unlucky victims. The list of risks is extensive. Accidents, alcohol, tobacco, and obesity top the list in terms of both prevalence and severity of outcome. On the other end of the spectrum, vaccines are deemed essentially safe, mad cow disease is too rare in humans to be a factor, mercury doesn't really affect most people, and pesticides have a minimal impact.

Risk attempts to reorient the reader. The authors would see dangers demystified. Their goal was to cut the public loose from hype and decontaminate us from prior misconceptions. But Cass Sunstein, a professor of law at the University of Chicago, distrusts authorities who approach us with a "we know what's best for you" attitude. In 2002, Sunstein published the book *Risk and Reason*, in which he suggested that it is not the expert or the official but the populist/consumer advocate who generally has our best interests at heart. Sunstein would likely distrust Ropeik and Gray's fear meters as simplistic and too easily politicized, preferring instead the judgment of the same consumer advocates that Ropeik and Gray might see as inaccurate.

According to Sunstein, "populists insist that the very characterization of risks involves no simple 'fact' . . . In the populist view . . . any judgment about risk is subjective . . . for populists, ordinary intuitions have normative force."

Like Ropeik and Gray, Sunstein also observed that information about risk was easily distorted, but unlike the authors of *Risk*, Sunstein generally blamed the government. He wrote, "Public officials know that they might be severely punished for downplaying a risk that is perceived as serious or for calling attention to a hazard that is perceived as trivial . . . to avoid charges of insensitivity . . . he [the public official] may make speeches and promote policies that convey deep concern about the very waste spill that he actually considers harmless."

The effective politician rides the waves from one created danger to the next: "Thus people might be fearful, for a time, about some risk—shark attacks, or air travel in the aftermath of a disaster—that produces no concern at all after a few months."

In the 2002 book *Risk Communication*, Drs. Granger Morgan, Baruch Fischhoff, and their coauthors suggested the need to integrate common beliefs with facts about risk. On the surface, this book seems to be an attempt to bring together the facts of Ropeik and Gray with the public intuition of Sunstein. The people who inform us need to consider "how the public intuitively thinks about the risks and . . . which aspects of the scientific literature actually matter to the public. Then those topics must be presented in a balanced, credible, and comprehensive manner."

If this declaration seems idealistic, it is because it relies on an agenda-free panel of public-minded experts. But learning to assess risk doesn't simply mean finding the right expert to listen to. We also have to take responsibility for our own fear meters. As Bruce Schneier, a world-respected security expert, wrote in his 2003 book *Beyond Fear*, "When you're living in fear, it's easy to let others make decisions for you. . . . To get beyond fear, you have to start thinking intelligently about the trade-offs you make. You have to start evaluating the risks you face."

Taking responsibility for our own fear meter sometimes means disregarding public pronouncements of risks, while at other times accepting them. But Schneier was concerned that we can too easily give up our freedom to a blanket authority that promises to handle our risk assessment for us but ultimately doesn't make us more secure, in part because this authority may tend to magnify threats. Like Sunstein, Schneier did not trust the usual experts and officials to advise us or protect us.

Wrote Schneier, "We are told that we are in graver danger than ever, and that we must change our lives in drastic and inconvenient ways in order to be secure. We are told that we must sacrifice privacy and anonymity and accept restrictions on our actions. We are told that the police need new far-reaching investigative powers, that domestic spying capabilities need to be instituted, and that we must spy on each other. . . . But the reality is that most of the changes we're being asked to endure won't result in good security. . . . Even in the worst neighborhoods, most people are safe.

It's hard to find a terrorist, kidnapper, bank robber, because there simply aren't that many in our society."

All the authors I have cited here are only partly right. We can't trust our risk experts, because their facts are amplified by the government, the media, and public advocates, each depending on different agendas. But this doesn't mean we can automatically trust our intuition either, which, as Gavin de Becker, author of *The Gift of Fear*, wrote, is too often "misinformed." Any resolution of this dichotomy between misinforming experts and misguided intuition must involve retraining in how to recognize danger.

Finding things to fear

On September 24, 2003, Anne Applebaum addressed the American terrain of worry in a column titled "Finding Things to Fear" in the *Washington Post*. She too was arguing against the wisdom of our unschooled intuition. She described how we have miscalculated risks in the post-9/11 world because of our continuing anxiety. "After Sept. 11, 2001, thousands of people in this country swore off airplanes and began driving cars, apparently believing that cars are safer. In fact, the number of deaths on U.S. highways in a typical year—more than 40,000—is more than double the number of people who have died in all commercial airplane accidents in the past forty years. To put it differently, the odds of being killed in a terrorist incident in 2002 were 1 in 9 million. In that same year, the odds of dying in a traffic accident were about 1 in 7,000. By taking the precaution of not flying, many people died."

Indeed, we are far safer in America, but we feel more afraid. We have thousands of safety devices, including smoke detectors, circuit breakers, and air bags. We are protected against everyday mishaps of all kinds. Yet if our fears aren't real, we invent them. The flow of information about risk has grown steadily during the same period of time that we have grown safer. Government officials, scientists, marketers, and the media use risk as a way to get attention. We tend to believe people who tell us that we are in danger. But when a warning such as an orange alert proves fallacious, we are slow to lose faith in the authority who has warned us. It takes several false warnings before we begin to question a source. By that time it is often too late, as our fear apparatus has already been triggered.

Recently, this apparatus has clearly been triggered by bird flu pandemic predictions and reports.

Conquering fear

For years, I have tried to help people handle their disease fears without knowing if I am succeeding or not. In studying the fear circuitry of the brain, I have now come to appreciate that teaching might not automatically lead to learning. Fear is a deep-rooted emotion, difficult for the brain to control. Sometimes its triggering can't be avoided. My daughter's experience with the Jacuzzi taught me that if fear is unlearned, it is because a new emotion replaces it. (She developed courage about returning to the bath.) This healing occurs at its own rate of speed, and a parent or a doctor often has little control over it.

To conquer fear we must return it to its primitive place as an instinct reserved for protecting us from true physical dangers. We must stop overpersonalizing it. We must resist those in the media and elsewhere who highlight the wrong dangers and hype the need to respond—making the threat seem even more real. We must regain our footing with regular sleep, regular meals, regular entertainment, regular exercise, and regular work. We must replace our unreal fears with real courage.

Tips for easing fear

I learned how to defeat fear from one patient, Joel Enrand. Enrand had an overriding terror of losing everything—his health, his job, his family—leading to depression, weight gain, high cholesterol, and elevated blood pressure. Most of all, with paralyzing middle-of-the-night bouts of sleepless fright, he was concerned about losing his mind. "You're not crazy," I reassured him. The tiny muscles around his eyes then relaxed. Enrand soon embarked on a program of his own design, willing himself to jog three miles a day before work, eat regularly, and limit himself to two cigars per week as his "one vice." After six months he sat, at ease, in my office. Seeing him like this, I knew I would recommend this "prescription" to other patients in a life crisis or suffering from fear of improbable risks such as bird flu.

"My courage is back, Doc," Enrand said. "Things were happening to me. I latched onto the worry. I could feel it, like it was real. It gripped me, and it grew."

"But you fought it?"

"Just by sticking to routines, rituals; they replaced the doubts little by little. When I saw I was getting my life back, I started to enjoy the routines." Enrand hesitated. "Most importantly," he said, "I'd always wanted to be a dad and I loved my son more than anything and I knew I was responsible for him. He needed me and I grew stronger by refusing to let go of him."

7

SARS

A vian flu isn't the first hyped respiratory virus from
Asia to dominate headlines in recent years. When, in
April 2003, SARS rose up to grab the media megaphone,
it set the standard by which all post-modern pandemic
false alarms ought to be measured.

SARS, or Severe Acute Respiratory Syndrome, brought
the panic over a potential infection to a new level. The
global health alert and travel advisories that were meant
to inhibit the dissemination of the virus—and that could
possibly do so under the right circumstances—also
spread virulent fear by word of mouth in this circum-
stance. Public health agencies raised the stakes, then
presumptively took credit for the resolution of the problem. The government sounded its note of preparedness,

wanting to seem proactive in another public panic situation where it was actually being reactive. The CDC, which had lost credibility with its bungling of the anthrax scare in October 2001, rallied publicly with SARS and quarantined entire sections of the planet in response to a virus that demonstrated seven thousand cases worldwide. The CDC and the World Health Organization (WHO) used fear to provoke compliance, talking about worst-case scenarios and viral mutations, and alarming the whole Western Hemisphere with a few cases that flew around a Toronto hotel.

But no one died of SARS in the United States in 2003, and people eventually grew tired of hearing about it. The CDC and the WHO had restricted travel to and from Asia and Toronto based on the assumption that air travel could allow an emerging contagion to spread more easily. This theory was neither proved nor disproved, though it certainly sounded convincing in the midst of the worldwide panic. But in fact, historically, isolating an afflicted patient has always been much more effective than quarantining a region. This principle had held true for plague, influenza, and many other contagious threats. People as they panic from an imposed quarantine can spread a bug. It is human nature to run away from perceived risk and human nature to make common mistakes when engaged in overinflated, hypervigilant activity. People who face heavy stigmatizing for being suspected disease carriers are likely to lose their common sense altogether.

Nevertheless, when the incidence of SARS died down (as many emerging viruses had done before it), the health organizations were quick to give credit to their worldwide advisory.

The chokehold

In early April 2003, President Bush granted Secretary of Health and Human Services Tommy Thompson the right to quarantine for SARS, thus giving a nudge to the trend that was spreading panic around the globe.

In its more than fifty years of existence, the WHO had never before issued a travel advisory or enacted a global surveillance network, as it did with SARS. In the United States, meanwhile, the CDC was publicly analyzing every conceivable case—another unprecedented reaction. SARS was a legitimate concern, and worldwide advisories certainly have a role in trying to contain disease, but the response was being carried to an extreme. By April, the virus had infected about two thousand people worldwide and killed fewer than one hundred, compared to the yearly average influenza death toll of thirty-six thousand in the United States alone.

What was going on medically? The answer was complex, since the SARS corona virus was a cousin to the common cold, which spreads easily via sneezing or even touch. But whereas the cold is countered by most people's immune systems, SARS was new, so our bodies hadn't yet had time to produce antibodies to it.

On the surface, a strong public health initiative of some kind seemed warranted.

As Julie Gerberding, the director of the CDC, pointed out in the *New England Journal of Medicine*, the cooperation of the international scientific community in identifying the corona virus as the culprit in a matter of weeks was very impressive. But Gerberding didn't stop with the scientists. She wrote: "Even more impressive than the speed of scientific discovery in the global SARS outbreak is the almost instantaneous communication and information exchange that has supported every aspect of the response."

But this was problematic. For the most part, the result of all this communication was global panic and economic shutdown that seemed way out of proportion to the real threat. Yes, today's communication system could certainly play an important role in identifying and containing an emerging disease. Yes, the WHO pressure on the Chinese medical authorities to take their heads out of the sand, identify patients, and isolate true cases was impressive. But beyond the historically proven method of isolating infected patients, it was difficult to tell how much air travel and the mobility now available to people—and their diseases—increased the mandate for regional embargo. This was an issue to be considered, but it wasn't an automatic justification for planet-wide sequestration.

The CDC appeared to be fully recovered from the public lambasting it had received over anthrax back in 2001. It had given itself a new face, with Gerberding as the new director giving speeches and press conferences at an unprecedented rate. SARS was a full-fledged international "bug du jour," with news and media coverage beyond those for any predecessor. The WHO, which had never gotten involved in global tracking strategies to this extent before, was weighing in heavily. In part this was due to improved technology, greater scientific cooperation, and an increased interest in tracking infectious agents because of concern over possible bioterrorism.

But neither organization was really used to the spotlight, and they weren't considering sufficiently how their reactions might be perceived by a fragile public. There was too much emphasis on public statements and not as much on serological testing and antiviral strategies. SARS needed to be cured with laboratory work, not press conferences. Panic over SARS was public health run amok. All the public posturing took SARS out of its proper context and contributed to a scare that ultimately did more harm than the virus itself.

By focusing only on the worst-case scenarios regarding the spread of SARS, the WHO and the CDC were in effect controlling the populace through fear. This helped to spread worldwide economic havoc—many estimates were that SARS cost over $30 billion to local economies worldwide. Toronto was cut off by the WHO travel advisory throughout much of April 2003. Chinatowns were deserted in all the major cities, and people around the world were stigmatizing anyone who came from an Asian country.

In contrast to the rest of Asia, Vietnam's careful and quiet isolating of suspected patients seemed to be behind its success in limiting the spread of the virus. Quarantining hospitals where SARS had spread to health care workers, or designating certain centers as "SARS hospitals," was at the upper limit of what seemed reasonable. Monitoring of traffic from countries where SARS had been diagnosed, or emphasizing careful precautions in such countries, was also reasonable but was not the same thing as frightening everyone who may have traveled there or who wanted to do so.

The problem with AIDS information in the 1980s had been the opposite kind of distortion: affected groups were marginalized, and the prevailing rhetoric had minimized the disease.

information, seeing the new disease in its context. At the time there were only thirty-five documented cases in the United States, and no one had died. We had to treat the perception that we could get SARS rather than any real risk of it. We needed to convert our uncertainty to a realistic understanding of our chances of getting the disease, which were extremely low for any given individual.

Overpersonalization of a minuscule risk spreads panic—and when people panic, they tend to take fewer precautions. How did a person know if he had SARS? The answer was that if he had a fever, muscle aches, and difficulty breathing, he didn't have SARS, but he probably had the flu.

A fear of Asians

The small waiting room in my office three blocks from New York University Medical Center was just as congested as the rest of New York, with patients sitting practically on top of one another. As with the subway, it felt as if germs here might spread more quickly than at other places, and I always half expected my patients to catch the bug their neighbor was harboring. But whether the risk of catching something from another patient was real or imagined, one thing was certain: the stress of living and working in the city made it seem so. Added to this mix, in the spring of 2003 we had the seemingly tangible risk of SARS. My waiting room was filled with patients, all brimming with the same question.

"Could I have SARS?" a patient blurted out. Unsolicited, an office secretary replied, "You must ask the doctor."

Meanwhile, the thirteen-inch television set in the

middle of the room was playing all SARS all the time and updating my patients on the virus every hour.

An Asian American architect, Mr. Ho, had come to see me for the first time. No one sat next to him in the waiting room, and when he coughed, the room emptied out altogether. In my examination room, Mr. Ho announced that he had just returned from Hong Kong. He traveled to China and Hong Kong on business every few weeks, but because of the effect of the SARS scare on the economy there, he had lost his latest architectural job and had had to come back. On the plane bringing him home, he said, no one would sit with him.

He came to me with a cough and symptoms of a cold, but no fever, no muscle aches, no difficulty breathing. Hearing this, I wanted to don a mask, but I put on gloves instead. My patient downplayed his symptoms, clearly realizing that I—the doctor—might be worried about SARS.

"It's just a cold," he said. "It was going away, then it came back a little. It's only a tickle."

Without saying the magic word, I reassured him that what he had sounded not like something sinister but like simple bronchitis.

I gave him an antibiotic and sent him home.

Afterward, I was suddenly nervous, thinking of my two young children. Doctors are not immune to worries about contagion. In my case, the concern didn't go away completely until I had taken a shower and irrationally washed away the psychological remnant of my fear. It was the same thing I used to do for AIDS in the 1980s, scrubbing my hands after every encounter with every potential AIDS patient.

A week later, Mr. Ho returned to the office with a smile

rather than a cough. During that week, the specter of SARS had spread through the world more rapidly than even the disease itself. Though not a single new case had been reported in our city, New Yorkers were increasingly frightened and increasingly wary.

Asia was more isolated than before, and Mr. Ho had no immediate prospect for work there. Back in New York, he thought people were taking into account his Asian features and avoiding him on the street. I could actually see this occurring in my waiting room, where the other patients now deliberately avoided not only him but anything he touched.

So why was Mr. Ho smiling? In my consultation room he confessed that he had actually been afraid he had SARS, but now that he knew he didn't, despite the fact that he was not working, he believed his future was bright.

SARS in New York City

New Yorkers are a nervous bunch to begin with, and our doctors are no exception. Most of us, doctors and patients alike, are medical Zeligs; like Woody Allen's character, we take on the symptoms and even the personality of the latest threat. The stress of living in an overcrowded city distorts perceptions in the direction of fear. The scientific literature analyzing the health of our city's residents shows that a disproportionately high percentage of New York teenagers suffer from eating disorders related to a higher level of stress. The same literature shows that proportionately more adults suffer from heart disease for the same reason. After studying this phenomenon, the journal *Psychosomatic Medicine* reported in 1999 that these conditions are due to the strain of life in New York itself.

New Yorkers try to compensate for the pressure we feel by paying more attention to our symptoms, to every itch and twinge, as if this vigilance might protect us from an ever-hostile environment. Our fear management is neurotic. Forever on the verge of panic, we seek out doctors more often and try to use elaborate health care safety nets to protect us from the ultimate free fall. The *Journal of Urban Health* in December 2002 described how New York's megacity has built an elaborate health system.

New York also has more media than anywhere else, and so we are more quickly saturated and prodded by the latest hype. We feel the strain earlier, but then we use our extensive safety net to become desensitized more quickly to the latest bug du jour, only to find ourselves right on the front lines of the next scare. It's a real roller-coaster ride.

In the era of SARS fear, we eventually developed a new sort of schtick. Though New Yorkers always cough and kvetch, I'd never heard so much nervous coughing before. We always seem to be on the verge of catching something, or if not actually catching something, at least complaining that we might. In the spring of 2003, each raspy breath seemed more significant, each sniffling acquaintance seemed ominously afflicted.

My office phone rang continually with respiratory complaints. I knew better than to counter these concerns with the bald statistic of zero deaths from SARS in the United States. I didn't want to appear to be downplaying serious potential risk, even if that risk was remote.

After a month of SARS hype, New Yorkers began building up an immunity to the fear.

According to the CDC, there were only two probable cases of SARS in New York City by May 2003, cases that ultimately turned out not to be SARS. So our respiratory filters joined our gas masks and our stash of antibiotics in our tiny closets.

SARS: When the smoke cleared

By July 2003, long after SARS had dropped off the headline news, it was determined that SARS had infected 8,400 people, killing 774 worldwide, with 33 probable U.S. cases and no deaths. After analyzing all the data from this outbreak, the WHO concluded that SARS is not spread easily through the air, but requires large respiratory droplets.

The Associated Press reported in October that fear over the possible return of SARS was so great in the United States that even if it didn't appear, the CDC expected emergency rooms to be swamped with suspected cases. They were concerned that doctors with limited SARS experience could confuse early SARS with the flu.

"Whether the virus comes back this winter or not, we will be dealing with SARS," said Dr. James Hughes, the director of the National Center for Infectious Diseases of the Centers for Disease Control and Prevention. "When people start showing up with respiratory diseases, physicians will be thinking of SARS. I can tell you we're more prepared than before," Hughes said. "I think the global community can handle SARS if it's handled appropriately. I think enough lessons have been learned" in the previous outbreak. Research on a vaccine and antiviral treatments were already under way.

As of February 2004, the outbreak still hadn't happened, with only three cases in Asia and none on the

North American continent. But the new viral bug du jour was flu, not SARS. Hughes was wrong. By early 2004, SARS seemed like a distant memory.

We really don't know what stopped the SARS outbreak in spring 2003. It may simply have run its course. It seems likely that hand washing and isolation of infected individuals helped, as the *New York Times* suggested in an editorial in early November 2003. But there was no direct evidence that the *Times* was right to conclude that "such tactics, buttressed by quarantines and restricted air travel, stopped the epidemic last time."

It clearly cost billions of dollars, and ironically, the *Times* editorial ended by reversing itself and cautioning the future use of aggressive tactics for SARS with a "recognition of the costs of any large-scale shutdown of normal activities."

But thanks to SARS hysteria, the apparatus was now in place for massive worldwide overreactions. If a disease died down, the health organizations and the media would take credit for its defeat without a true scientific study to prove they were right. If a disease seemed to get out of hand, the news media would continue to report it without ever acknowledging the way they—the media— were instantly altering the public's sense of risk. In China, Zhong Nanshan, a scientist who had dealt with the first SARS outbreak, had a more practical plan. He urged people just to avoid spitting in public and eating wild animals.

8

THE OTHER FLU

In early December 2003, TV and radio across the country relentlessly covered the "flu outbreak." Practicing physicians appeared on multiple stations to respond to sudden concerns.

Marvin Scott, the WB11 weekend anchor in New York, a man with a classic, sonorous TV voice, a square chin, and the pockmarks of a veteran newsman, seemed insulted that I didn't recognize him.

He rushed into my pale blue consultation room on the cold winter afternoon of December 10 with his cameraman and his agenda ready. Some children had died, and he seemed to want me to say that all parents should be concerned. His first question was about what parents should be doing to protect their kids.

I cautioned that parents shouldn't overreact. The

sniffles your child complained of might well be the common cold, whereas flu tends to manifest itself with sudden high fevers, chills, severe muscle aches, and headaches.

"Eleven children have died in one state," he said dramatically. "The number is climbing. Is this an epidemic?"

Scott's questions wouldn't go on TV, only my answers, wrapped together in a sixty-second sound bite. It was important for me to not utter a single phrase that might play into the hype. I told him that young deaths were clearly a tragedy, but not an epidemic.

"Should parents be keeping their kids out of schools?"

"Parents should be encouraging hand washing and should always keep sick kids at home. But flu is far from widespread enough to consider closing schools."

"What should parents do?"

"All day long my office telephone rings with nervous parents wanting to get flu shots for their kids."

"What do you tell them?"

"I tell parents that flu shots are not strictly necessary unless their kids have asthma or another chronic illness."

By the time he left my office, Marvin Scott seemed calmer. He had a hype bias, but he was open to fresh facts. It was true that children were dying—twenty or thirty by December 12. How many the total number would be wasn't yet known. Still, the danger to any of us or our kids remained far less than it seemed.

Flu perception was far worse than the reality. Here is what I told my patients: schools closed for blizzards, not flurries. Our 2003 flu was a flurry, not a storm. Since we were on a heightened flu alert, we were likely to mistake every cough or sneeze for that bad bug, but doctors could usually tell whether their patients were overreacting or actually required immediate attention.

The yearly outbreak

Before 2003, flu was an underappreciated ho-hum domestic killer. It was traditionally robbed of the attention it deserved by the latest bug du jour. Thirty-six thousand people died of the flu in the United States yearly, but many didn't get the vaccine who should have. In previous years, the flu simply didn't worry enough people.

In the fall of 2003, all of that changed overnight, as talking-head doctors told TV viewers why they should worry: it was an earlier season then usual, a worse flu bug than usual, and the vaccine didn't really cover this flu, which appeared to be a killer of children. But the true epidemic was not from flu virus but flu fear.

The CDC and the WHO, now assuming the go-to position with every potential contagion, once again seized the media megaphone as soon as a few children started to die of flu in late November. I received hundreds of phone calls from healthy patients demanding the flu shot, a vaccine that was rapidly becoming scarce. One healthy young patient, whom I hadn't seen in over two years, called urgently for a shot because her sister was afraid to let her visit the newborn baby two days hence without one. I was able to slow her down only by pointing out that two days wasn't sufficient time for the shot to work. Even at the height of the concern, no one knew whether the flu season was going to be any worse than in prior years, when the media had paid little attention.

Scares one group, kills another

While 70 to 80 million had received the flu vaccine the year before in the United States, another 70 million were advised to receive it but didn't. Health care workers, those with respiratory or chronic illnesses, pregnant women, the elderly, and anyone who might come in close contact with the flu are on the CDC's recommended list to be vaccinated. Influenza affects 20 percent of the U.S. population in a given year, and over two hundred thousand people are hospitalized on average. The yearly flu vaccine is generally considered to be 40 to 60 percent effective at preventing the flu.

The CDC reported 85 million doses of the vaccine available in 2003, as the vaccine manufacturers based their year's supply on the previous year's usage. In 2002, they had had to discard over 10 million unused doses, and they weren't about to repeat that costly move in 2003. This way of determining supply inevitably led to a shortage in a year when the devastating deaths were broadcast and hyped by the media. By early December 2003, people were clamoring for the vaccine even as supplies of it ran short.

The WHO has a global influenza surveillance system involving 112 regional influenza centers. These centers study the early patterns of the year's flu in Asia and South America. The WHO then makes its best guess of what the predominant strains would be here and makes up the vaccine for the most common serotypes. Unfortunately in 2003, the Fujian strain of influenza A, which was going to cause a lot of the havoc, wasn't included in the vaccine because of difficulty getting it to reproduce in the culture medium.

Flu history

The flu is an ancient scourge, tracing its origins back at least to the days of Hippocrates, who recorded an outbreak of an illness that began with a cough, followed by pneumonia and other symptoms, at Perinthus in ancient Greece in 400 B.C.

There were several pandemics (disease spreading widely over a large region) in the eighteenth century, but the most massive outbreak ever occurred in 1918, a topic which I've covered here in chapter 3. As I've also mentioned, in 1968, the Hong Kong flu killed 700,000 people worldwide, and this may well have set us up for the swine flu panic of 1976, when the outbreak was minuscule, but the rush vaccination program led to over a thousand cases of Guillain-Barré syndrome, a form of paralysis. Luckily, the current version of the flu vaccine—even though antiquated—is much safer than the rush vaccine used in 1976.

Influenza experts agree that another pandemic is likely to happen at some point. Some epidemiological models project that in industrialized countries alone, the next such scourge is likely to result in 57 million to 132 million outpatient visits, 1 million to 2.3 million hospitalizations, and 280,000 to 650,000 deaths over less than two years, or at least five to ten times what we tend to experience in an average flu year. However, these models don't take into sufficient account that a quickly developed vaccine may slow spread. A "herd immunity" may also have occurred from prior vaccination or exposure to similar flu strains. These models also overlook the effect of modern medical treatments that prevent complications and decrease the severity of the illness. Communication can help control or spread a pandemic virus, depending on whether the operative term is restraint or panic.

As with previous pandemics, the impact of the next flu blight is likely to be greatest in developing countries where health care resources are strained and the general population is weakened by poor health and nutrition. So the WHO and the CDC work at expanding the flu surveillance and containment network.

One reason for the potential panic out of proportion to the risk is that it is almost impossible to predict when this pandemic might occur. The event occurs only about once in fifty years, but the more we see it discussed in the media, the more we personalize the uncertainty, convincing ourselves irrationally that every year will be the year.

The making of a bug du jour

Before 2003, flu was underappreciated. It was a widely held, yet poorly acted upon, public health perception that we needed more vaccinations, more isolation of those who were sick, and more hand washing. When I first saw flu hit the headlines, I hoped that the sudden attention would shed light on these basic precautions. Unfortunately, the flu scare of 2003 did not necessarily lead to proper prevention, but as with all bugs du jour, it involved significant expense.

By mid-December, influenza had completed its transition from ho-hum killer to whopping bug du jour. By December 12, it was all over the Internet that the flu had spread to all fifty states. Flu did this every year, though usually not until January, and in previous years most people who didn't have the flu paid little attention.

Dr. Julie Gerberding, the director of the CDC, was the official spokesperson for the flu, as she had been for every bug du jour since anthrax. She seemed to have gained insight since SARS and was now attempting to be the voice of reason.

But once again, she addressed the phenomenon without acknowledging that the perception of a scourge was a media creation. "I think what we're seeing is a natural response to concerns about a serious flu season," she said on December 12 on NBC's *Today* show.

"But we also need to remember that for almost everyone, flu is not such a serious disease. We don't need to panic or assume that the worst-case scenario is going to happen to everyone. Most of us will get through this fine," she said.

Meanwhile, thousands all over the country lined up for flu shots wherever they could find them, mostly in response to the spreading fear. The federal government announced that it was scrambling to ship 100,000 adult vaccine doses to combat the shortages, hoping to head off what they felt could become one of the worst flu outbreaks in years, and 150,000 child vaccines were expected in January. The government, by wanting to show that it was preparing, helped spread the sense of urgency. Around the country, schools began to shut down. Emergency rooms were filling with sick children, many of whom just had colds. Doctors' offices were forced to turn away droves of people seeking flu shots. An Internet poll of 30,000 people reported 57 percent who said nothing more could be done, but 43 percent who felt this vaccine didn't offer adequate protection. Both of the vaccine manufacturers, Chiron and Aventis, had shipped their entire supply, though Aventis had set aside 250,000 doses that it was giving to the CDC for distribution. The CDC also managed to procure 375,000 more doses from Great Britain.

Gerberding said the CDC was recommending doctors give high-risk groups top priority for shots. Despite the severity of the early outbreak, health experts were still not able to predict just how bad the flu season would be! The season could still just be peaking early.

Surprise ending

In mid-December, the government continued its rush to find extra vaccine doses (as it had in 1976) to help quell the panic it had helped to create. Dr. Walt Orenstein, the director of the CDC's National Immunization Program, fanned the fear flames by announcing that this was still looking like a bad flu season for children. Ninety-two children die in an average flu year. It was still too early to tell whether this number would be exceeded in the 2003–2004 season, though parents everywhere, fueled by media hype, continued to act as if it would.

The buzz among doctors was that it was highly unusual for healthy children to be dying from this flu. This unscientific observation, though it concerned only a few dozen patients nationwide, helped to spread the panic. Then suddenly, the news media stopped reporting on the flu. The CDC was just starting to use the word "epidemic" when the media showed its attention deficit and veered away.

The flu willies of 2003 were actually treated inadvertently by the capture of Saddam Hussein. On the morning of December 14, 2003, Paul Bremer, the U.S. administrator of Iraq, announced, "Ladies and gentlemen, we got him." The message was that because this evil man had been captured, the world was by definition much safer. The news media broadcast this central message for more than a week, to the exclusion of any fear messages. The famous video footage of Saddam's mouth yielding to a tongue depressor replaced all images of sick children lying on hospital gurneys. The sense of relief we felt carried over to many aspects of our lives. We went through a "feeling safe" week and lumped the flu into the group of things we were automatically feeling safer from. Flu was displaced from the headlines, so we stopped thinking about it. It briefly seemed as if nothing deadly at all could take place now that the world's worst monster was in custody.

Seeing safety in these simplistic terms—that the world, with a broken-down Saddam snaked out of his hole, was suddenly safe where it hadn't been before—was a distortion, a perversion of the facts. It was as if the military's accomplishment was somehow a cure for all our ills, and for all potential ills, including influenza. In reality, we were no more and no less susceptible to the risk of this year's flu than the day before Saddam's capture when the flu was all over the Internet, the Associated Press, and the top of the cable shows' news cycles 24/7. The sudden transition from palpable panic to utter disregard served to underline the extent to which our fears were manipulated and were ultimately unrelated to actual dangers.

"There is no firm line dividing what's an epidemic and what's not an epidemic," Gerberding emphasized on December 19, when people were no longer listening. "But I think when you look at maps with widespread activity in thirty-six states, we regard it from a common-sense perspective as an epidemic." The CDC said its emergency operations center had been up and running for two weeks, but rather than be alarmed by this announcement, the media barely covered it, and those people who knew about it ignored it. Anthrax, West Nile virus, and SARS had driven people wild with worry while actually killing fewer than fifty people combined in the Western Hemisphere. Influenza, a proven killer of thirty-six thousand people per year in the United States alone, was first ignored, then obsessed over, and then ignored again. If there was a silver lining to all this fear-induced distortion, it was that increased public awareness might help the health care system contain the flu in the future—provided that some awareness of the real disease remained once the roving eye of the media had moved on.

The sequel: Flu vaccine 2004

In August 2004, Dr. Gerberding of the CDC stated that "the time to be complacent about the flu is over."

Dr. Anthony Fauci, the head of the National Institute for Allergy and Infectious Diseases, said on CNN, "There is really a full-court press going on now to develop" flu vaccines that protect against many strains of the virus, including the current bird flu.

Fauci, a world leader in infectious diseases, spoke with his usual gravitas, which unfortunately gave the impression that an outbreak was looming.

Without evidence, and with minimal risk, the cycle of worry was restarting, and it was using as an unwitting mouthpiece one of our most dedicated scientists.

The golden shot

In fall 2004, the year's first flu-related death came not from the disease, but from an elderly woman who fell while waiting in line for the vaccine. This unfortunate event added to the annals of illness, where panic has always killed far more than the disease that caused it. With the announcement that 50 million influenza vaccines from the manufacturer Chiron wouldn't be available in the United States because of possible contamination, the CDC was put in an instant quandary, its credibility once again damaged. From pushing the yearly flu vaccine accelerator pedal, urging everyone to get a shot, they suddenly had to slam on the brakes, their reassurances, of course, sounding hollow.

"Take a deep breath, this is not an emergency," Dr. Gerberding said, trying to change her persona instantly from apocalyptic to therapeutic.

The sudden panic of people with fear memory from the prior year's flu, primed for the shot but now with nowhere to go for it, was likely to cause a stampede of shot seekers. The CDC had helped create a new monster. The frantic healthy folks could easily beat out the elderly short-of-breath patients who really need the vaccine to protect them from serious illness. The CDC's attempts to referee this problem were bound to be ineffective.

The whole flu-shot fiasco was an example of inadequate preparation coupled with overinflated expectation and a fear of going without. One of the main reasons that a shortage like this could occur is that drug manufacturers are not eager to produce vaccines in the first place. Vaccines are costly. Without a patent to uphold high prices, the profit margins for generic vaccines are narrow. As I've mentioned in previous chapters, the chicken-egg culture medium still being used to produce vaccines needs to be replaced by the latest in genetic engineering, but the changeover involves another billion-dollar expense.

Forget altruism, or concern for patients—they are

not essential parts of the drug company equation. Drug companies are not eager to make a product they can't make a lot of money on. The only workable solution to prevent the panic of a sudden shortage is for the government to step in and support and subsidize the manufacture of this vaccine. The plan of buying back unused vaccines isn't sufficient. It is far more important to ensure production of an adequate number of vaccines in the first place.

Instead, Congress approved only half of the $100 million requested in 2003 to develop better flu vaccines and improve the distribution system.

The British did not end up with the same kind of shortage despite the Chiron manufacturing disaster on their soil, because they rely on a diversity of manufacturers, and the government purchases the entire supply itself, so the public needn't worry.

In contrast, in late October 2004, U.S. health authorities began scrambling to make up some of our lost doses from other countries' stockpiles. Canada had 2 million doses of surplus vaccine to make available for U.S. use, according to David Butler-Jones, Canada's public health officer. But there was difficulty licensing them for use in the United States in time for the 2004 flu season. There were six manufacturers in the world who produced 200 million doses for other nations in 2004, while only two, Chiron and Aventis, were entirely responsible for our 100 million doses.

In Germany, there is not the same urgent push for the flu vaccine. A study carried out by Berlin's Robert Koch Institute in November 2003 showed that the average influenza vaccination rate in Germany is only 23.7

percent. The numbers are somewhat higher for those over sixty, but Germans overall appear to be less fearful of the flu than we are here in the United States, despite the fact that a comparable percentage, five to eight thousand people, die of the flu in Germany every year. In 2004, Germany had 20 million doses of the vaccine available for its use, and didn't report a shortage.

The difference in flu fear between countries may be cultural. A ninety-year-old woman I know in northern Germany not only doesn't believe in flu shots, but she believes in an ice-cold shower in the morning and open windows in the bedrooms without heat even in the winter. Yet, she is no more irrational than those who believe the flu shot is a panacea.

In the United States, the rush for the 2004 shot was based on fear, not on medical science. The well-publicized scarcity created a sudden sense of need. And by the time the smoke cleared in January from yet another mild flu season, there was an embarrassing surplus of shots that people no longer wanted. By this time, the attention of the news media was diverted to the deadly tsunami on the other side of the world, and no one was thinking about the flu except for the few who had it.

Bioterror instead of flu

Instead of preparing for the flu, our government has been busy spending billions of dollars stockpiling millions of doses of anthrax vaccine (with no use for it in the foreseeable future) and over two hundred thousand doses of smallpox vaccine (without a single case occurring here since 1949). These actions have been taken at least partly so that Homeland Security can look as if it takes the threat of biological agents seriously. A bioterror attack would likely affect only hundreds or, worst case, thousands at once, yet the expensive preparations are for millions of potential victims.

Bioport makes the only current anthrax vaccine, an unwieldy six-dose process that many military recruits have complained gives them a flulike syndrome. But fearing an anthrax attack since 2001, the U.S. government has contracted with this company for 75 million doses of the vaccine. Since the vaccine is perishable, and there is no anthrax here, most of what is produced is thrown away. Similarly, panicked over smallpox in 2002 and 2003, the government purchased 291,400 doses of the antiquated live virus vaccines, discarding 90 percent of them due to fear of side effects and lack of need.

Meanwhile, the CDC has determined that at least 185 million Americans could benefit from flu vaccine, either because they are at risk of getting very sick or are in close contact with those who are. Yet with the shortage in 2004, the available supply of flu vaccine that year was only about 54 million doses. The CDC was soon begging Aventis to produce more, but the company made available only 1 million additional doses. Was this all it could make, or all it would make? No one I spoke to at the manufacturer was able to provide an answer.

Instead of the government spending all its vaccine money on the production of nearly useless bioterror vaccines, a more substantial flu subsidy could lead to the consistent availability of at least 100 million doses, which would calm nerves and perhaps even save lives.

Who gets the shot?

The waiting room of my office was filling with frantic healthy patients who had come in without appointments, all yearning for the coveted 2004 vaccine. My phone was ringing incessantly with the same question. Does he have it yet? I told most callers no, though I had scrounged and begged my usual supplier for five vials, enough for fifty of my sickest patients. But I didn't tell anyone this, trying to avoid a stampede. The flu vaccine is useful, but it is not the key to good health.

Plenty of people make it through the winter safely without it. Most of my patients would do fine without a shot in 2004, but knowing that there was a scarcity had clouded people's reason. I offered my elderly and chronically ill patients a vaccine against pneumonia, which I had in ample supply, but even when they took it, they hardly seemed reassured by my observation that it was often pneumonia that made flu patients the sickest. The lucky few who did get the flu shot didn't flinch from the needle puncture, but sighed with an almost palpable relief as the protective serum surged into their muscle. For the others I stressed hand washing and isolating those with the flu, but driven by the news, frantic shot seekers ignored this calmer perspective.

In 2004 I was bound by public health authorities to give the vaccine I did have to the very old, the very young, the very sick, pregnant women, and health care workers. This was a good policy, because I had so little.

Within this policy, I set my own sub-policy—to give it only to those who already had an appointment and the sickest who called in. Like many other doctors, I had set aside office visits in the early fall to give these vaccinations, and I had neither enough appointments left nor flu shots for the panicked many.

I reassured those who weren't at great risk, and I saved some of my fifty shots for my office staff, my pregnant wife, and my elderly parents. For the first time in years I was compelled to ration supplies, which caused me to properly consider which patients were most susceptible to serious infection.

I declined to charge higher rates for giving an older patient the shot. An unethical doctor could make money in a hurry under these panicked circumstances, but he could also go to jail for Medicare fraud.

One night, I made a rare house call, taking a vial to Long Island. One of my chronically ill patients was an old friend who was housebound with a bad leg, and I drove out to see him. He was relieved to see the syringe, the alcohol pad, and, especially, the vial. But afterward, as I was getting ready to leave, he stopped me. "Can my wife have one too?"

On cue, she was standing in the doorway, a woman in her early fifties, eager for a flu shot, but not qualifying for one. "No," I said. "I can lose my license for giving this out to the wrong people. Think of the people who are really at risk." She was ready to give up, but he wasn't. "Can't you make an exception?" he pleaded.

The tension was so great that I actually dropped the precious vial. I thought I heard it crack when it hit the floor, and I felt certain I had broken it. They both peered at me anxiously as I bent to pick up the magic elixir and retrieved it as it was rolling away.

Luckily, the contents were intact.

"Okay," I said nervously. "Maybe she qualifies. You're at high risk, and she's a close contact. I can give her a shot."

They sighed and thanked me repeatedly, more than they had the last time he was treated successfully for pneumonia.

I felt good, like a medical Robin Hood. It was only afterward, driving home, that I thought of my dwindling supply and considered a fragile wheezy patient with an office appointment a few weeks hence who wouldn't be able to get a shot because of the one I'd just given away.

9

DO WE KNOW A PANDEMIC WHEN WE SEE ONE? AIDS VERSUS BIRD FLU

By the end of January 2004, it was clear that the human flu for the season had peaked and petered out. Ironically, it was actually a mild flu season. This was fortuitous, because the flu shots given across America in the fall of 2003 were for a slightly different strain than we actually experienced, and the Centers for Disease Control (CDC) reported that the year's mismatched vaccine had not succeeded in diminishing flu symptoms. The disease had simply run its yearly course, despite the panic about shortages.

By January 24, 2004, though, we suddenly began hearing about the avian flu H5N1, the new potential bug du jour. The *New York Times* provided extensive front-page coverage, creating a sense of immediacy and sweeping importance: "The announcement, made by the Thai government on Friday, has deepened fears of a global epidemic if the virus combines with another that can be transmitted from person to person."

The Thai government had reportedly suppressed the information about the sick chickens for weeks in order to protect its chicken industry, as China had suppressed information about patients sick with SARS the year before to protect tourism. Once uncovered, this suppression stoked fears.

The City of New York Department of Health and Mental Hygiene issued a new advisory on January 28, 2004, alerting health care providers to widespread outbreaks of avian influenza A in domestic poultry and wild birds in ten countries in Asia, where by the beginning of February it had also infected over twenty humans among bird handlers and their relatives, killing fourteen. If you'd traveled to Asia recently and returned to New York with respiratory symptoms, you were being asked to report to the health department. If this public health alert expanded, panic could result.

Birds, as a disease carrier, have the potential to scare us. Like tiny Lyme-ridden deer ticks and buzzing West Nile–carrying mosquitoes, they could be anywhere and everywhere. Worse, we can actually see these birds, flocking everywhere we go, ominously. But in terms of a bird flu affecting us, as I've explained in previous chapters, human-to-human transmission is extremely unlikely unless a mutation to the virus occurs. Thousands of avian flu viruses never make that journey to humans.

A *New York Times* editorial on January 30, 2004, acknowledged that "the threat to Americans is virtually nonexistent," but went on to state that "health officials are rushing to prepare a seed virus for vaccine production, but full-scale production could take months." The problem with this sort of rhetoric was that while professing calm, it unintentionally spread fear.

Not yet on our shores

Despite the fact that not a single infected bird had escaped the Asian continent, Lee Jong-Wook, director general of the World Health Organization (WHO), had also helped to prime the pump toward chicken phobia on January 28, 2004, with the statement, "This is a serious global threat to human health."

In the meantime, back in 2004 I stubbornly believed that as an American bug du jour, the avian flu would not make the same impact that the others did as long as it didn't jump the ocean.

I was wrong, as I will show. In the fall of 2005, in the wake of Hurricane Katrina, avian flu became a full-scale bug du jour simply by virtue of its potential.

Over in Asia, the virus was already creating havoc back at the beginning of 2004, bringing up memories of SARS even if the victims this time around were birds, with few human deaths. Over one hundred million chickens, crows, and ducks died across Asia, mostly from government-ordered slaughters rather than from the disease. It was difficult to know how much bird carnage was necessary in order to control the disease. But in the process, a second virus, fear, spread, as vivid television and newspaper images of unprotected people throwing dead chickens into pits or stuffing them live into sacks was enough to spread local hysteria and threaten economic shutdown, as it did with SARS.

Here in the United States, thousands of chickens were

being killed in Delaware for another, unrelated bird flu that was not as sinister and did not sound the public health alarm (though it led China to ban our chickens, just as Japan was banning our beef because of a single case of mad cow disease).

No scientific study had been done to determine how many chickens needed to be killed to prevent the significant spread of a bird flu even among just birds.

A key factor keeping Americans from full-blown bird panic in early 2004 was that we weren't ready yet to consider another influenza. We were desensitized to flu viruses for the time being after the yearly human flu-vaccine shortage scare. By late 2005, bird flu came at us like a swooping bird, as if it were unrelated to the yearly flu.

Still, the groundwork to scare us in late 2005 was laid in early 2004. The *Wall Street Journal* provided a stirring front page headline on January 28, 2004: "Bird-flu Outbreak Revives Concerns Stirred by SARS."

This article described the poor public health conditions that were bound to provoke fear: "Animals and people living in close and sometimes unsanitary quarters; poor regulation of livestock; and ill-equipped public-health workers hamstrung by local governments so anxious to avoid panic and economic pain that their actions border on a coverup."

Dr. Julie Gerberding of the CDC was quoted in the article: "This could be a very serious problem if the epidemic in Asia is not contained." Which epidemic was that? Perhaps she meant to say the chicken epidemic.

The *Journal* backed up its front-page story with another story, titled "Scientists Rush to Create Vaccine for Bird Flu—Just in Case."

What was all this rushing about?

The *Journal* article provided the answer in a box insert: "Some experts worry the virus could morph into a human superflu, as in the pandemic of 1918–1920." Here was scary 1918, invoked again. And the ultimate drama: "We have to think about the potential for a significant population die-off," said Dr. David Fedson, formerly of the vaccine maker Aventis.

Was Dr. Fedson being mercenary? Fear could put pressure on the government to push the panic button, stockpiling massive amounts of vaccine that would have to be discarded if not used in three years.

Vaccines are perishable, fear is not.

Bird flu's draconian potential

John Barry, author of *The Great Influenza: The Epic Story of the Deadliest Plague in History*, was right about the need for preparation and information, as long as this information was well reasoned. He wrote in an op-ed in *USA Today* on February 10, 2004: "A public information effort must be launched to convince people of the threat and heighten cooperation. From the perspectives of public health and national security, the bird flu in Asia already should have the full attention of every government in the world."

Cooperation among scientists and governments is crucial to developing a strategy of prevention for any serious disease, including avian influenza. But it is just as crucial, while raising public awareness to gain support for needed programs, to also learn ways to inform without alarming. Once fear or worry is provoked, it is difficult for humans to process information without over-personalizing and magnifying the threat. The economic and psychological cost of fear is far too great for it to have a role in anything other than the most imminent of threats.

In early 2004, it was the television rather than the print media that seemed to be sounding a cautionary note. The cable news coverage of the bird flu didn't appear to be as extensive as what the *New York Times* or the *Wall Street Journal* provided. A producer at CNN told me that they didn't "want to appear to be sensationalizing the story."

The brief concern with bird flu in 2004 had died by February, replaced by domestic concerns. All this would soon change, however, in the fall of 2005, when the cocked heads, wild eyes, and ruby red lips of countless chickens paraded across the screens of America's living rooms.

By 2004, great scientists studying the worldwide laboratory were becoming too interested in the latest bug in the news. With publicized contagions, our public health experts easily put aside the rigor of their training and fell into a trap of hype. Public health had gotten too entangled with the media, and infectious disease experts had begun automatically using the media megaphone to broadcast their message.

It is true that avian flu, if it morphs into a human-to-human virus, could cause another worldwide pandemic, perhaps as deadly as the one in 1918. But many viruses and bacteria have the potential to harm; it is up to public health agencies to distinguish between potential and looming. Disease information is contextual—it is never an all-or-nothing situation as portrayed in the news.

On into 2004 and 2005, the CDC continued their public demonstrations of vigilance for any and all health threats. Led by Dr. Gerberding, they responded quickly with multiple press conferences to each new perceived threat.

Our public health experts continued to use words like "vigilance" and "rush to a vaccine" when describing a needed reaction to the bird flu. These were the same words they used for SARS and before that, smallpox, and before that, West Nile virus. These aren't informative words; they don't give us any special insight into a health risk, and they don't help us to discern a potential from an ongoing risk. Beyond misdirecting us away from looming health risks like obesity and smoking, public health sound bites may also provide wrong information. Clearly, an epidemiological need to track an emerging disease before it gets out of hand is not the same thing as saying the entire public is already at risk.

Part of the problem is that lab scientists who have never been trained in public speaking are suddenly clipped and quoted in the newspapers or thrust onto the television screens and asked to provide three-minute descriptions of something they may have spent a lifetime studying. There is an understood pressure to make it sound important or exciting. This pressure leads easily to distortion and overstatement.

So we stockpiled millions of doses of smallpox vaccine in preparation for an attack that didn't come, to protect us against a bug that hadn't made anyone sick here since 1949. When the moment of fear and worry was upon us, our public health experts made us worry more. Unfortunately, in the case of smallpox, these vaccines were perishable, and since hardly anyone agreed to take them, this meant that millions of dollars' worth of prevention then had to be thrown away.

Unlike the talking points for a TV sound bite, the criteria for publishing a paper in a top scientific journal are stiff. You have to study the requisite number of patients to make sure the study is statistically significant. Often studies are double-blinded, which means you can't know the results ahead of time. There is a need for careful controls, and all data has to be checked and rechecked. No self-respecting scientist would have it any other way. Why should the criteria be less stringent when scientists inform the public about these same health issues?

The bird flu scare of 2005

We didn't hear much about bird flu throughout most of 2004 or 2005 even as it continued its march through the domestic birds of Asia. Americans tend to pay little attention to health issues overseas until those issues are seen as directly threatening us.

Then in early October 2005, in the wake of Hurricane Katrina, two further studies on the structure of the 1918 Spanish flu molecule were published in the respected journals *Nature* and *Science*, and Gina Kolata revealed in a front-page article of the *New York Times* on October 6, 2005, that "the 1918 influenza virus, the cause of one of history's most deadly epidemics, has been reconstructed and found to be a bird flu that jumped directly to humans, two teams of federal and university scientists announced yesterday. It was the culmination of work that began a decade ago and involved fishing tiny fragments of the 1918 virus from snippets of lung tissue from two soldiers and an Alaskan woman who died in the 1918 pandemic."

This article appeared to state that the 1918 virus had just been discovered to be a bird flu that had jumped to humans, a fact that had actually been known for many years. And each study over the past ten years had shown a bit more of the virus's structure and determined how it made the jump; the latest two studies were just a furthering of prior work.

Unfortunately, this article and others like it helped to fuel the concern that something was in the offing with the current H5N1 bird flu. The sense of immediacy and discovery in the media invited the comparison to not only the 1918 virus, but to the pandemic itself, despite the significant difference in the structure of the current virus versus the 1918 virus as well as fundamental differences in health care and communication resources in 1918 as opposed to now.

On the same day, on the front page of the *Wall Street Journal*, the following story appeared: "U.S. Sees Need to Better Prepare Against Avian Flu." Bernard Wysocki Jr. wrote, "Amid growing concerns about bird flu spreading to humans, the Bush administration says it plans to bolster vaccine production in the U.S., purchase huge quantities of antiviral drugs and lay out a detailed system to coordinate federal, state, and local response efforts to a pandemic."

It was clear that avian influenza was a problem. Unfortunately, amid a quickly growing consensus that some bird flu would mutate and cause the next pandemic (how severe and when no one could say), all the media attention carried with it an implied urgency that made everyone think the moment for a dreaded mutation causing a pandemic was near. But there was simply no evidence for this.

Further, though the sudden public interest in bird flu

seemed bound to push the Bush administration to designate funds for pandemic preparedness, which was in itself a very good thing, there was also a key question of where the money was going to be spent. Stockpiles of perishable Tamiflu and the new bird flu vaccine were bound to be an expensive part of any plan that would be wasted unless a pandemic occurred within a narrow time frame. And though no health expert could fault the government for preparing for a huge disaster no matter how slight the risk at any given point in time, the sudden spotlight on the issue also made many people think personal stockpiles were in order.

But personal stockpiles are problematic, because it is then up to the patient when to take a drug that has no current indication, has side effects, and can breed resistance, rendering it less useful.

Money better spent would be used for establishing an integrated network of public health responders worldwide, nationally, and locally. Best of all for bird flu would be a worldwide effort to combat the disease in birds.

Earlier the same week, President Bush began to speak publicly for the first time about his own concerns about a possible flu pandemic. He mentioned using the military to quarantine entire cities if necessary, an instant fear message. His intention was clear—to show that in the event of another national disaster of the scope of Hurricane Katrina or much greater, this time the federal government would be prepared to respond in time.

Bush was quoted widely as saying he got his idea and concern about a pandemic from reading John Barry's excellent account of the 1918 Spanish flu pandemic, *The Great Influenza: The Epic Story of the Deadliest Plague in History*, and some pundits would comment wryly that the president might have been better off reading Barry's other master work, about the great Mississippi flood of 1927, in advance of Hurricane Katrina.

George J. Annas, chairman of the Department of Health Law, Bioethics and Human Rights at Boston University School of Public Health, wrote a stirring op-ed in the *Boston Globe* on October 8, 2005, calling Bush's idea of using the military in a flu pandemic "dangerous" and a misreading of Barry's book. Annas pointed out that although quarantine was used successfully in 1918 on the island of American Samoa, Barry in his afterword suggested a comprehensive national plan, not a show of force to deal with a future influenza pandemic. But Annas also disagreed with Barry's subsequent use of the words "extreme quarantine" and wrote that "planning for 'brutal' or 'extreme' quarantine of large numbers or areas of the United States would create more problems than it could solve." Annas went on to describe convincingly the limitations of quarantine. "First, historically mass quarantines of healthy people who may have been exposed to a pathogen have never worked to control a pandemic, and have almost always done more harm than good because they usually involve vicious discrimination against classes of people (like immigrants or Asians) who are seen as 'diseased' and dangerous . . . quarantine is no magic bullet . . . quarantine and isolation are often falsely equated, but the former involves people who are well, the latter people who are sick. Sick people should be treated, but we don't need the military to force treatment. . . . Sending soldiers to quarantine large numbers of people will most likely create panic, and cause people to flee (and spread disease), as it did in China where a rumor during the SARS epidemic that Beijing would be quarantined led to 250,000 people fleeing the city that night. . . . The real public health challenge will be shortages of health care personnel, hospital beds, and medicine. . . . And effective action against any flu virus demands its early identification, and the quick development, manufacture, and distribution of a vaccine and treatment modalities. . . . It is a misreading of history that a lesson from 1918 is to militarize mass quarantine to contain the flu. And neither medicine nor public health are what they were in 1918; having public health rely on mass quarantine today is like having our military rely on trench warfare in Iraq."

Annas concluded by presenting a clear vision of how the feds should proceed in developing a strategy of prevention and containment toward a worst-case scenario flu pandemic. "National flu policy will be determined by national politics. In World War I, as Barry recounts, this policy demanded that there be no public criticism of the federal government. That policy was a disaster, and did prevent many effective public health actions. . . . Public health in the 21st century should be federally directed, but effective public health policy must be based on trust, not fear of the public."

The only downside of Annas's piece was that it contributed to a growing dialogue of implied imminence about the next 1918 "Blue Death." This was clearly, at least to me, a public health and media creation. Luckily, a week following the publication of the two studies in *Nature* and *Science*, several newspapers, including the *New York Times* and the *Washington Post*, published articles that tried to show the broader perspective. The *Times*, in a front-page article by Denise Grady headlined "The Danger Is Clear, But Not Present," wisely quoted virologists who pointed out that although avian influenza would certainly cause another pandemic at some point, the culprit might well not be the H5N1 virus. And when a pandemic did occur, modern medicine, public health efforts, and worldwide communication and cooperation could keep another Spanish flu–type devastation from occurring.

In *Newsday* on October 12, 2005, health writer Delthia Ricks reported that the National Institutes of Allergy and Infectious Diseases was testing a bird flu vaccine in senior citizens, and that people were "lining up" to get it. I was quoted in the article expressing caution about the potential usefulness of the vaccine. "If bird flu does mutate, we have no idea whether it will mutate into a form in which the current vaccine is even useful . . . it's not as if the virus doesn't have tendencies that are deadly, but right now it's mostly killing birds, and before it can routinely kill people, it has to mutate." Also in this article, Dr. Len Horovitz, a pulmonary specialist at Lenox Hill Hospital in Manhattan, said he believed clinically testing a vaccine was important, though in the end, it might not mutate. "There certainly is a lot of hysteria, and right now, I think we need to put things into perspective."

How to prepare?

In the newly created *Weekend Wall Street Journal*, on October 22–23, 2005, an editorial took on the issue of preparedness for avian influenza. The central point of the editorial was to analyze how ill prepared we were, no matter what the actual risk, to make the vaccines necessary to protect us. "Whatever the risk, some good will come out of this public alarm if we use it as an opportunity to understand why the U.S. is now so poorly armed to cope with a deadly flu outbreak. The reason is that our political class has spent the last 30 years driving the vaccine industry out of business with its own virus of overregulation, price controls, litigation, and intellectual-property abuse."

The *Journal* was right to consider that vaccine manufacturing was so hamstrung by political and legal concerns that it avoided upgrading to crucial new technologies. As the editorial eloquently stated, "The industry has revolutionary new technologies—reverse genetics and mammalian cell culture—that would dramatically reduce the time and cost of development."

But the *Journal* was wrong to ultimately conclude that the solution was less government involvement rather than more. Private industry could certainly not be counted on to work without regulation, be trusted to ensure its own safety, while at the same time be relied upon to produce an adequate supply at a time of sudden crisis.

When at the end of October 2005, President Bush proposed a $7.1 billion expenditure to Congress for pandemic preparedness, he seemed to understand just this point—that the government needed to be directly involved with vaccine manufacture to ensure the upgraded technology. In fact, his plan called for $2.7 billion for just this purpose, while he also stressed the need for legislative reform in order to protect the drug makers against lawsuits.

A *New York Times* editorial, "The Perplexing Pandemic Flu Plan," published on November 20, 2005, championed this aspect of the Bush plan, but pointed out that its implementation was vague.

Other critics of the plan pointed to its lack of funding to the state and local health agencies, which would be crucial in coordinating health care in the event of a pandemic of any kind. And far less than $1 billion was designated for fighting the disease in birds, where if it was controlled, the ultimate risk to humans would be far less. Others criticized the more that $2 billion that went for stockpiling of bird flu vaccines and Tamiflu. Some said it was too little and too slow (only 20 million doses of vaccine, not to be stockpiled until 2009), while others, myself included, pointed out that these stockpiles, as with those for bioterror protection, would be wasted if not used for a worst-case scenario because their shelf life was only about three years. Plus, if the bird virus mutated, it was hard to know if either the current vaccine or Tamiflu would be effective.

Quarantine whom?

On November 22, 2005, the *New York Times* reported that the CDC had opened ten new quarantine stations at major ports of entry into the United States, with the intention of opening several more, with a close eye on avian flu. This was occurring in advance of any possible mutation, whereas in the past, quarantine stations have been useful during worldwide outbreaks to help prevent the spread of yellow fever (1878) and cholera (1892) into the country. The program was essentially disbanded in the 1970s with the eradication of smallpox but has been renewed in recent years in response to concerns about bioterror and SARS.

Quarantine, though useful during an outbreak of an emerging disease, has been limited historically because of fear. People whose movements are restricted tend to panic, and panic causes people to take fewer precautions and thereby spread more disease. Isolation of infected individuals has therefore been more effective a technique historically than sequestering entire regions.

A problem with considering quarantine now is that the bird flu in its current form has not been transmitted human to human, and setting up quarantine centers with bird flu in mind would seem to send the message that a mutation is imminent. Such a message would add to the unnecessary fear.

We already have a pandemic

Not to minimize the human sickness and death of the bird handlers in China, but while the world ramped up its obsession with avian influenza in 2005, AIDS continued to infect more than 40 million people in the world, the number having doubled in a decade. According to a UN report, AIDS killed approximately 3.1 million in 2005, with more than 5 million new cases. According to Peter Piot, executive director of the UN AIDS program, the 5 million new cases is the most in a year since the beginning of the epidemic.

Asia accounted for roughly 20 percent or 8.3 million of the 40 million cases worldwide. While being chastised over their handling of bird flu, in the meantime, the UN report indicated that HIV had been found in all provinces of China, mainly due to prostitution and the use of needles by illegal drug users. In China, 60 percent of those infected with HIV contracted the infection through drug use. Only about twenty thousand people were receiving HIV antiretroviral treatment in twenty-eight provinces.

AIDS remorselessly advanced in 2005, infecting nine people every minute, destroying families, societies, and economies throughout the world but most prominently in sub-Saharan Africa, with 3 million new HIV infections, almost two-thirds of the world's total new cases. The steepest increase took place in eastern Europe and central Asia, where the rate of HIV infection rose 25 percent to 1.6 million.

On the rare positive front with AIDS, in Kenya, HIV rates declined 3 percent over the past five years, partly due to education campaigns promoting HIV testing and routine condom use.

The standard HIV prevention strategy has maintained that the key to success is increasing access to treatment with antiretroviral drugs. Once patients are aware that there is treatment available, they are more inclined to get tested; and once they know they are HIV positive, they can be counseled and informed to try to avoid further spread.

According to Lee Jong-Wook, WHO director general, "Treatment availability provides a powerful incentive for governments to support and individuals to seek out HIV prevention information and voluntary counseling and testing."

Unfortunately, the world's eyes are focused elsewhere. AIDS scared us more here in the West in the 1980s when we knew less about it and had little idea how to treat it. Now that current therapies save thousands of lives from HIV here every year, we have too little interest in making sure that these treatments are spread around the world to the neediest places. Since western medicine has driven the response to infections that have emerged in Africa and Asia, the fact that we here in the United States are now more afraid of the distant threat of bird flu than the ever-present threat of AIDS is relevant.

Only approximately 1 million people were taking antiretroviral drugs in low- and middle-income countries by June 2005, 2 million below the WHO target.

Only one in ten of those infected with HIV in the world has received treatment. More money and more medicine are clearly needed. It wouldn't be fair to say that these resources are being diverted to theoretical risks such as the current avian influenza; on the other hand, the world health community doesn't have unlimited financial or educational means.

Here in the Western world there were 1.2 million cases of HIV in 2005. The United States exceeded 1 million infected for the first time in 2003. The United States and Western Europe, the only regions in the world where antiretroviral treatment is readily available, have reported 65,000 new HIV infections in the past year, in part because of people who have come here from countries with more serious AIDS epidemics. Of course, the lack of emphasis on condom distribution and use leads to a snowballing effect of the disease.

The movement of HIV from countries with lesser resources to the countries with abundant treatments underlines the need to make HIV disease a far greater worldwide priority. Global travel and global communications have created a global responsibility—to stamp out disease beyond our borders.

Is bird flu the next AIDS?

I began my medical internship in 1985, in the heart of the AIDS era. Just a few years before, when I was in medical school, AIDS cases were nonexistent. By the time I had my M.D. degree, people were dying of the mystery virus everywhere.

At the beginning of the process, I had no sense that this disease would become rampant, and by the end, in 1985, as I saw patients ravaged and quickly dying, I had no hope that AIDS would one day soon be transformed by medical science into a treatable, if still uncontained, epidemic.

Many scientists and journalists have used the rampant, unpredicted, underappreciated HIV explosion as justification for responding to bird flu in advance. This is partly justified—at least the understanding that an epidemic can get out of hand faster than the worldwide health community can respond to control it.

But how many emerging diseases should we extend the AIDS model to, and how often can we afford to be wrong—at what expense? Public health doesn't have a great batting average over the past few years, warning us about mad cow disease, anthrax, smallpox, West Nile virus, and SARS. None of these has progressed into the realm of killer diseases dominated by AIDS, tuberculosis, and malaria. Yet all were touted and promoted as the "next AIDS."

In 2003, SARS, like the current bird flu, was expected to rifle through the world community because of the zero immunity we had to it. Surely the worldwide health response, including quarantine, played a role in snuffing SARS, but the larger reality was that SARS petered out on its own, that it wasn't as infectious a virus as we thought it was.

Similarly, the H5N1 bird virus has the potential to harm us and kill millions, but as with the killer prion proteins of mad cow disease, we are currently protected by a species barrier. Hence, with many millions of birds dead from the virus as well as culled in our attempts to control it, the numbers are minuscule for humans—over 130 known symptomatic infections, with 70 deaths to date.

The billion-dollar question: Is there a way for public health experts to predict which disease will be the next AIDS, or do we have to keep getting it wrong until we get it right? The answer is that scientists do have clues. Instead of scaring the public about the H5N1 bird flu virus, it is far more prudent to analyze it in the laboratory, where studies show that it is a deadly, ever-changing virus that is still several changes away from being able to affect us routinely. Probably the best use of AIDS-caliber resources with the current bird flu virus would be to continue to target birds rather than humans.

The HIV virus is blood-borne and is easily destroyed in the environment, but when it gets into a human host, it targets the immune system, the very system of cells that we use to protect ourselves. It is not a surprise that HIV is such an effective killer. It is more a surprise to me, and a testament to the reach of modern science, that effective treatments have been developed for it.

The H5N1 virus is far different from AIDS. It is heartier in the environment, but it doesn't pass easily to humans. It affects the breathing system of birds, choking them off with infection. It cannot become the next AIDS (or something far worse than AIDS) without mutating. Even if it does mutate, keep in mind that influenza viruses kill mostly by weakening the host and allowing serious secondary infections such as pneumonia to take over. As with AIDS, we can treat these infections, provided we extend our technology to enough places.

The chances of this worst-case scenario occurring are small, but as Michael Leavitt, the secretary of the Department of Health and Human Services has said, "It is not zero."

10

PERSPECTIVES

When my office finally got its supply of flu vaccine this year, it was later than usual but in plenty of time for flu season, which usually doesn't start until late December. Yet being offered a regular flu shot didn't seem to reassure most of my patients.

One typical Thursday five patients begged for prescriptions for Tamiflu, and two asked for a shot of bird flu vaccine, which doesn't yet exist.

The last patient of the day muttered as he was leaving, "Bird flu is going to get us all this year."

The difficulty with informing the public about a potential pandemic from a doctor's point of view is that the uncertainty about when or if it could occur breeds fear. Scared people overpersonalize the news just as they overinterpret their potential for illness, and their worries increase.

The greatest problem among my patients right now

isn't bird flu; it is fear of bird flu. The greatest risk of an epidemic is of a fear epidemic.

What are we all so afraid of?

Bird flu is indeed a threat—especially if you have wings.

Most of my patients understand this, and they know just as well as I do that there is no bird flu in the United States. What scares them is the possibility of a pandemic. It's remote, but it's real—the hardest kind of risk to put in perspective.

Why the overreaction in this case? Worst-case news reports, including constant comparisons to the terrifying flu pandemic of 1918, have scared my patients out of all proportion.

Projections of numbers ill or dead in a worst-case pandemic are unsettling. Michael Leavitt, the secretary of the Department of Health and Human Services, announced on December 5, 2005, that the United States is preparing for a possible 92 million Americans sick within sixteen weeks, with schools closed and businesses disrupted. It is hardly reassuring to hear such staggering numbers along with a vague caveat like "just in case."

But as I've emphasized throughout this book, even if we accept the Spanish flu scenario, health conditions in 1918 were far worse in most of the world than they are now. Today's media and public health reach could be a useful tool to aid compliance. We also have our top scientists and epidemiologists tracking this avian flu, which was not the case in 1918 prior to the essential mutation.

But instead of this reassuring information, our TV screens continually project images of beleaguered Asians and stricken birds. We attach ourselves voyeuristically to the news, reported by sincere people who often are overly afraid themselves. We all too easily jump to presume that a near impossibility is now suddenly inevitable.

Grabbing the media megaphone

If Americans are afraid of avian flu now, imagine what will happen if a single scrawny, flu-ridden migratory bird somehow manages to reach our shores. Problematic as it would be from a medical point of view, it would be like a lit match to the fuel tank of our stored-up fears. Our economy would take a big hit as people became afraid to come here, and our poultry would be shunned around the world. We would also become prey to fearmongers, who would no doubt claim that their product or their leadership was the only thing that could protect us.

This is how fear works, how the fear epidemic—as opposed to a flu pandemic—spreads. Fear is supposed to be our warning system against imminent dangers, but as a deep-rooted emotion, it interferes with our ability to make sound judgments. And if anything is contagious right now, it's judgment clouded by fear.

Fearmongers are having a field day lumping bird flu together with other deadly disasters. Dr. Shigeru Omi, the World Health Organization's regional director for the Western Pacific, recently said, "Even if you control avian flu, the next one is coming. . . . I think it is similar to tsunamis and earthquakes . . . we do not know when." Comparisons to tsunamis scare a lot of people unnecessarily.

Unfortunately, public health alarms are sounded too often and too soon. SARS was something to be taken seriously, but the real lessons of SARS, smallpox, West Nile virus, anthrax, and mad cow disease weren't learned by our leaders—that potential health threats are more effectively examined in the laboratory than at a news conference.

It is true that AIDS taught us that we need to look seriously at emerging threats before they spread. But AIDS still kills nearly 3 million people every year in the world, tuberculosis nearly 2 million, and malaria about 1 million. We would be far better off using our personal fear radar against these diseases than against a bird disease that's still off in the distance.

The unseen microbe

Instead of the constant grandstanding, consideration should be paid to using public warnings for the health threats with the greatest probability of occurrence and the greatest likelihood of affecting many. It is too easy to focus on the risks of a sinister-sounding killer like a deadly mad cow prion or a bird virus that historians revere.

Unseen, deadly microbes have a certain dark fascination. Mysterious descriptions conjure fear well beyond our actual risk. Meanwhile, it is heart disease and stroke that kill over a million Americans a year, automobiles that injure 50 million and kill 1 million worldwide, and hurricanes that drive us from our homes.

Why are we so scared?

People are voyeuristic about illness, and we all personalize it. So when you hear that someone is sick, you wonder if it's going to be you next. When someone you know has been diagnosed with cancer, for example, it is a common impulse to get checked yourself. In the age of instantly refreshable Internet news sites, twenty-four-hour cable TV, and news cycles that restart every five seconds, it's easy to misuse our voyeuristic tendencies and feel falsely alarmed.

We humans have the ability to inform our fear mechanism by assessing risk. But when we hear about bird flu pandemics, we don't know how to respond, because the information is too abstract. We can be smarter than animals, but we're often not.

Dr. Elizabeth Phelps, a neuroscientist at New York University, has examined how the brain responds to envisioned threats. Using highly sensitive MRI scans, she discovered that the brain's fear center (the amygdala) can be activated in response to dangers a person merely observes. "When you are watching it and you are told that it is going to happen to you, it causes the same robust response by the amygdala as if you actually experience it yourself," Phelps said. She has also studied the safety signals that our brains use to turn off fear; it turns out the brain's wiring heavily favors the "on" switch.

That leaves us humans forever in the position of trying to turn off a response that often shouldn't have been turned on in the first place. Since our fear radar doesn't discriminate, we release stress hormones unnecessarily, readying for a crisis that doesn't come. Heart rates and blood pressure increase, we breathe harder, and like a car that revs constantly at high speed, we are more likely to break down. What bothers me most as a physician is that I see my patients being harmed, and there's little I can do to stop it. Fear is infectious, and the fear of bird flu has become particularly virulent. There is a vaccine for this fear: it is called information mixed with perspective. Since there is a shortage of this vaccine, fear has begun to spread throughout my community and yours. That is a chilling foretaste of the horror of a true epidemic.

BIBLIOGRAPHY

INTRODUCTION

———. "U.S. Scours Files to Trace the Source of Mad Cow Case." *New York Times,* Dec. 24, 2003.

Corradi, Juan E., Patricia Weiss Fagen, and Manuel Antonio Garreton. *Fear at the Edge: State Terror and Resistance in Latin America.* Berkeley: University of California Press, 1992.

Grady, Denise. "U.S. Issues Safety Rules to Protect Food against Mad Cow Disease." *New York Times,* Dec. 31, 2003.

Hitchcock, Alfred, and Sidney Gottlieb (editor). *Hitchcock on Hitchcock: Selected Writings and Interviews.* Berkeley: University of California Press, reprint edition, Nov. 1997.

Kertesz, Imre. *Fateless.* Evanston, Ill.: Northwestern University Press, 1992.

McNeil, Donald G. "Mad Cow Disease in the United States: The Overview; Mad Cow Case Leads Government to Consider Greater Meat Testing." *New York Times,* Dec. 26, 2003.

Melamed, Samueal. "Association of Fear of Terror with Low-Grade Inflammation among Apparently Healthy Employed Adults." *Psychosomatic Medicine* 66, no. 4 (Aug. 2004): 484–91.

Merkin, Daphne. "The Way We Live Now: 8-15-04; Terror-Filled." *New York Times Magazine,* Aug. 15, 2004.

New York Times. "Faulty Levees" (editorial). Sept. 22, 2005.

Reinberg, Steven. "1918 Influenza Genes Similar to Modern Bird Flu." *HealthDay,* Oct. 5, 2005, quoted Dr. Julie Gerberding of the Centers for Disease Control and Prevention, "It's not a matter of if but when."

Russert, Tim. *Meet the Press,* NBC, Nov. 20, 2005.

Schlosser, Eric. "The Cow Jumped over the U.S.D.A." *New York Times,* Jan. 2, 2003.

Spencer, Jane, and Cynthia Crossen. "Why Do Americans Believe Danger Lurks Everywhere?" *Wall Street Journal,* Apr. 24, 2003.

Steinberg, Jonathan S., et al. "Increased Incidence of Life-Threatening Ventricular Arrhythmias in Implantable Defibrillator Patients after the World Trade Center Attack." *Journal of the American College of Cardiology* 44, no. 6 (Sept. 15, 2004): 1261–4.

Talan, Jamie. "Mad Cow Scare, Fears Confirmed, More Questions Than Answers." *Newsday*, Dec. 26, 2003.

Tierno, Philip M. *The Secret Life of Germs: Observations and Lessons from a Microbe Hunter*. New York: Pocket Books, 2001.

USAID. "Statistics on AIDS, malaria, tuberculosis." www.usaid.gov/ our_work/global_health/ home/News/ghachievements.html (accessed Dec. 5, 2005).

Wald, Matthew L., and Eric Lichtblau. "U.S. Is Examining a Mad Cow Case, First in Country." *New York Times*, Dec. 24, 2003.

Whelan, Elizabeth. "Mad Cow Kerfuffle." *New York Sun*, Dec. 26, 2003.

CHAPTER 1. BIRD FLU BASICS

Alderman, Michael. "The Flu's Second Front." *New York Times*, Op-ed, Nov. 30, 2005.

Balicer, R. D., M. Huerta, and I. Grotto. "Tackling the Next Influenza Pandemic." *British Medical Journal* 328 (2004): 1391–92.

Barker, W. H., and Mullooly, J. P. "Impact of Epidemic Type A Influenza in a Defined Adult Population." *American Journal of Epidemiology* 112 (1980): 798–811.

Billings, Molly. "The Influenza Pandemic of 1918." http://www .stanford.edu/group/virus/uda/. June 1997; modified Feb. 2005.

Bowman, Lee. "A Look at Bush's Plan to Fight Bird Flu." Scripps Howard News Service, Nov. 1, 2005.

Cauchemez, S., F. Carrat, C. Viboud, A. J. Valleron, and P. Y. Boelle. "A Bayesian MCMC Approach to Study Transmission of Influenza: Application to Household Longitudinal Data." *Statistics in Medicine* 23 (2004): 3469–87.

Centers for Disease Control and Prevention. Avian influenza facts. http://www.cdc.gov/flu/avian/gen-info/facts.htm (accessed Dec. 5, 2005).

———. "Influenza Prevention and Control." http://www.cdc.gov/ ncidod/diseases/flu/fluvirus.htm.

Council on Foreign Relations. www.cfr.org/publication/9280/ council_on_foreign_relations_conference_on_the_global_threat_of_ pandemic_inf (accesssed Dec. 5, 2005).

Department of Health. Influenza Immunisation: Chief Medical Officer's update. 1997. [cited 2005 Mar 1]. http://www.dh.gov.uk/assetRoot/ 04/01/35/74/04013574.pdf.

Fedson, D. S. "Pandemic Influenza and the Global Vaccine Supply." *Clinical Infectious Diseases*. 36 (2003): 1552–61.

Fleming, D., J. Charlton, and A. McCormick "The Population at Risk in Relation to Influenza Immunisation Policy in England and Wales." *Health Trends* 29 (1997): 42–7.

Fock, R., H. Bergmann, H. Bußmann, G. Fell, E.-J. Finke, U. Koch, et al. "Influenza Pandemic: Preparedness Planning in Germany." *Eurosurveillance* 7 (2002): 1–5.

Health Canada. Canadian Pandemic Influenza Plan, 2004. [cited 2005 Mar 1]. http://www.phac-aspc.gc.ca/cpip-pclcpi/.

"The Influenza Epidemic in England and Wales 1957–58." *Reports on Public Health and Medical Subjects*, no. 100. London: Her Majesty's Stationery Office; 1960.

Jefferson, T., D. Rivette, A. Rivetti, M. Rudin, C. Di Pietrantonj, and V. Demicheli. "Efficacy and Effectiveness of Influenza Vaccines in Elderly People: A Systematic Review." *The Lancet* 366 (2005): 1165–74.

Johnson, N. P., and J. Mueller. "Updating the Accounts: Global Mortality of the 1918–1920 'Spanish' Influenza Pandemic." *Bulletin of the History of Medicine* 76 (2002): 105–15.

Kiso, M., K. Mitamura, Y. Sakai-Tagawa, K. Shiraishi, C. Kawakami, K. Kimura, et al. "Resistant Influenza A Viruses in Children Treated with Oseltamivir: Descriptive Study." *The Lancet* 364 (2004): 759–65.

Longini, I. M., M. E. Halloran, A. Nizam, and Y. Yang. "Containing Pandemic Influenza with Antiviral Agents." *American Journal of Epidemiology* 159 (2004): 623–33.

Mayo Clinic. "Bird Flu: Avian Influenza." http://www.mayoclinic.com/health/birdflu/DS00566/DSECTION=8&.

Mann, P. G., M. S. Pereira, J. W. Smith, R. J. Hart, and W. O. Williams. "A Five-Year Study of Influenza in Families." Joint Public Health Laboratory Service/Royal College of General Practitioners Working Group. *Journal of Hygiene* (Lond). 87 (1981): 191–200.

McKimm-Breschkin, J., T. Trivedi, A. Hampson, A. Hay, A. Klimov, M. Tashiro, et al. "Neuraminidase Sequence Analysis and Susceptibilities of Influenza Virus Clinical Isolates to Zanamivir and Oseltamivir." *Antimicrobial Agents and Chemotherapy* 47 (2003): 2264–72.

Medline Plus. Influenza information. http://www.nlm.nih.gov/medlineplus/flu.html.

Meltzer, M. I., N. J. Cox, and K. Fukuda. "The Economic Impact of Pandemic Influenza in the United States: Priorities for Intervention." *Emerging Infectious Diseases* 5 (1999): 659–71.

Mills, C. E., J. M. Robins, and M. Lipsitch. "Transmissibility of 1918 Pandemic Influenza." *Nature* 432 (2004): 904–6.

Monto, A. S. "Influenza: Quantifying Morbidity and Mortality." *American Journal of Medicine* 82 (1987): 20–6.

National Institute for Clinical Excellence. "Guidance on the Use of Zanamivir, Oseltamivir and Amantadine for the Treatment of Influenza." www.nice.org.uk/pdf/58_Flu_fullguidance.pdf (2005).

Nguyen-Van-Tam, J. S., and A. W. Hampson. "The Epidemiology and Clinical Impact of Pandemic Influenza." *Vaccine* 21 (2003): 1762–8.

Nguyen-Van-Tam, J. S., S. A. Leach, B. Cooper, R. Gani, N. J. Goddard, J. M. Watson, et al. "Tackling the Next Influenza Pandemic: Ring Prophylaxis May Prove Useful Early On, but Is Unlikely to Be Effective or Practical to Implement Once the Pandemic Is Established." *British Medical Journal* B 22 July 2004. [Cited 2005 Mar 1]. http://bmj.bmjjournals.com/cgi/eletters/328/7453/1391#68042.

Pang, X., Z. Zu, F. Xu, J. Guo, X. Gong, D. Liu, et al. "Evaluation of Control Measures Implemented in the Severe Acute Respiratory Syndrome Outbreak in Beijing, 2003." *Journal of the American Medical Association* 290 (2003): 3215–21.

Patriarca, P. A., and N. J. Cox. "Influenza Pandemic Preparedness Plan for the United States." *Journal of Infectious Diseases* 1997;176 (Suppl 1): S4–7.

Reports on public health and medical subjects no. 4: report on the pandemic of influenza 1918–19. London: Her Majesty's Stationery Office; 1920.

Stiver, G. "The Treatment of Influenza with Antiviral Drugs." *Canadian Medical Association Journal* 168 (2003): 49–57.

Taylor, M. P. "Influenza 1968–1970 Incidence in General Practice Based on a Population Survey." *Journal of the Royal College of General Practitioners* 21 (1971): 17–22.

United Kingdom Department of Health. UK pandemic influenza contingency plan. March 2005 [cited 2005 Mar 1]. http://www.dh.gov.uk/assetRoot/04/10/44/37/04104437.pdf.

United States Department of Health and Human Services. "Pandemic Flu." www.pandemicflu.gov.

United States Food and Drug Administration. "Q and A on Bird Flu and Food Safety." www.cfsan.fda.gov/~dms/avfluqa.html.

Van Genugten, M. L., M. L. Heijnen, and J. C. Jager. "Pandemic Influenza and Healthcare Demand in the Netherlands: Scenario Analysis." *Emerging Infectious Diseases* 9 (2003): 531–8.

Wainright, P. O., M. L. Perdue, M. Brugh, and C. W. Beard. "Amantadine Resistance among Hemagglutinin Subtype 5 Strains of Avian Influenza Virus." *Avian Diseases* 35 (1991): 31–9.

Webby, R. J., and R. G. Webster. "Are We Ready for Pandemic Influenza?" *Science* 302 (2003): 1519–22.

World Health Organization. www.who.int/en/.

————. "Influenza pandemic plan: The role of WHO and guidelines for national and regional planning." Geneva: The World Health Organization, 1999.

CHAPTER 2. THE HISTORY OF BIRD FLU

Barry, John M. *The Great Influenza: The Epic Story of the Deadliest Plague in History.* New York: Viking Books, 2004.

British Medical Journal. July 13, 1918, p. 39; Oct. 19, 1918, pp. 439–40; Nov. 2, 1918, pp. 494–96, 503; Nov. 16, 1918, p. 546; Nov. 23, 1918, p. 573; Nov. 30, 1918, p. 620; Dec. 21, 1918, p. 694.

Brown, David. "It All Started in Kansas." *Washington Post Weekly Edition,* Mar. 23–30, 1992; vol 9, no. 21.

Collins, S., and J. Lehman. "Excess Deaths from Influenza and Pneumonia and from Important Chronic Disease during Epidemic Periods 1918–1951." Public Health Monographs no. 10, 1953.

Committee on the Atmosphere and Man. "Causes of Geographical Variation in the Influenza Epidemic." *National Research Council Bulletin,* July 1923, vol. 6, no. 34.

Crawford, Richard. *Stranger Than Fiction: Vignettes of San Diego History.* San Diego, Calif.: San Diego Historical Society, 1995. http://edweb.sdsu.edu/sdhs/stranger/flu.htm.

Crosby, Alfred. *America's Forgotten Pandemic: The Influenza of 1918.* Cambridge, England, and New York: Cambridge University Press, 1989.

Deseret News. "On the Eve of Peace in WWI Influenza Cast Shadow of Death." http://www.desnews.com/cen/hst/01260133.htm.

Grist, N. R. "A Letter from Camp Devens 1918." *British Medical Journal,* Dec. 22–29, 1979.

Henig, Robin Marantz. "Flu Pandemic: Once and Future Menace. " *New York Times Magazine,* Nov. 19, 1992.

Hoagg, Jesse. "The Influenza Virus Unveiled." *The Experience* , 1997, http://www.the-experience.com/issue2/flu.htm.

Hoehling, A. A. *The Great Epidemic.* Boston: Little Brown and Company, 1961.

Hughes, Sally Smith. *The Virus: A History of the Concept.* New York: Heinemann Educational Books Ltd., 1977.

Journal of the American Medical Association. Oct. 5, 1918, pp. 1136–1137; Oct. 12, 1918, p. 1220; Dec. 7, 1918, pp. 1928–9, 1935; Dec. 14, 1918, p. 2015; Dec. 21, 1918, pp. 2068–73; Dec. 28, 1918, pp. 2154, 2174–5; Jan. 4, 1919, pp. 31–34; Jan. 11, 1919, pp. 155-59; Jan. 18, 1919, p. 188; Jan. 25, 1919, p. 268; Mar. 1, 1919, p. 640; Apr. 12, 1919, pp. 1056–58.

Knox, Richard. "Deadly 1918 Flu Virus Could Reappear, Report Says." *Boston Globe*, Mar. 21, 1997, www.globe.com.

Nature. "Avian Influenza." http://www.nature.com/nature/focus/avianflu/timeline.html.

New York State Department of Health. "A Special Report on the Mortality from Influenza in New York State during the Epidemic of 1918–19," 1923.

Starr, Isaac. "Influenza in 1918: Recollections of the Epidemic in Philadelphia," *Annals of Internal Medicine* 85 (1976): 516–18.

Taubenberger, Jeffery, et al. "Initial Genetic Characterization of the 1918 'Spanish' Influenza Virus." *Science* 275 (1997): 1793–96.

Tice, D. J. "Flu Deaths Rivaled, Ran alongside World War I." *Pioneer Planet*, Mar. 10, 1997.

United States Census Bureau. "Special Tables of Mortality from Influenza and Pneumonia in Indiana, Kansas, and Philadelphia, Pa., September 1 to December 1, 1918," 1920.

CHAPTER 3. SPANISH FLU VERSUS SWINE FLU

"An Influenza Outbreak at Fort Dix Had Been Caused by the Swine-Type Influenza A Virus." www.hsph.harvard.edu/Organizations/DDIL/swineflu.htmlat.

Alvord, E. C. Jr. "Swine Influenza Vaccine and Guillain-Barré Syndrome: Lies, Damn Lies, and . . ." *Archives of Neurology* 43, no. 10 (1986): 979–82.

Beghi, E., L. T. Kurland, D. W. Mulder, and W. C. Wiederholt. "Guillain-Barré Syndrome: Clinicoepidemiologic Features and Effect of Influenza Vaccine." *Archives of Neurology* 42, no. 11 (1985): 1053–57.

Benenson, A. S., ed. *Control of Communicable Diseases Manual*. 16th ed. Washington: American Public Health Association, 1995.

Bregman, D. J. "Guillain-Barré Syndrome: Its Epidemiology and Associations with Influenza Vaccination." *Annals of Neurology* 9, supplement (1981): 31–38.

Breman, J. G., and N. S. Hayner. "Guillain-Barré Syndrome and Its Relationship to Swine Influenza Vaccination in Michigan, 1976–77." *American Journal of Epidemiology* 119, no. 6 (1984): 880–89.

Brown, D. "A Shot in the Dark: Swine Flu's Vaccine Lessons." *Washington Post*, May 27, 2002.

Crosby, Alfred W. Jr. *Epidemic and Peace: 1918*. Westport: Greenwood Press, 1976.

Greenstreet, R. "Adjustment of Rates of Guillain-Barré Syndrome among Recipients of Swine Flu Vaccine, 1976–77." *Journal of the Royal Society of Medicine* 76, no. 7 (1983): 620–21.

Greenstreet, R. L. "Estimation of the Probability That Guillain-Barré Syndrome Was Caused by the Swine Flu Vaccine: US Experience (1976–77)." *Medicine, Science and the Law* 24, no. 1 (1984): 61–67.

Hoehling, A. A. *The Great Epidemic.* Boston: Little, Brown and Company, 1961.

Hogg, J. E., D. E. Kobrin, and B. S. Schoenberg. "The Guillain-Barré Syndrome: Epidemiologic and Clinical Features." *Journal of Chronic Disease* 32, no. 3 (1979): 227–31.

Kolata, Gina. *Flu:The Story of the Great Influenza Pandemic of 1918 and the Search for the Virus That Caused It.* New York: Simon & Schuster, 1999.

Kurland, L. T., W. C. Wiederholt, J. W. Kirkpatrick, H. G. Potter, and P. Armstrong. "Swine Influenza Vaccine and Guillain-Barré Syndrome. Epidemic or Artifact?" *Archives of Neurology* 42, no. 11 (1985): 1089–92.

Laitin, Elissa A., and Elise M. Pelletier. "The Influenza A/New Jersey (Swine Flu) Vaccine and Guillain-Barré Syndrome: The Arguments for a Causal Association." Harvard School of Public Health, 1997, http://www.hsph.harvard.edu/Organizations/DDIL/swineflu.html.

Langmuir, A. D. "Guillain-Barré Syndrome: The Swine Influenza Virus Vaccine Incident in the United States of America, 1976–77: Preliminary Communication." *Journal of the Royal Society of Medicine* 72, no. 19 (1979): 660–69.

Langmuir, A. D., D. J. Bregman, L. T. Kurland, N. Nathanson, and M. Victor. "An Epidemiologic and Clinical Evaluation of Guillain-Barré Syndrome Reported in Association with the Administration of Swine Influenza Vaccines." *American Journal of Epidemiology* 119, no. 6 (1984): 841–79.

Mantel, N. "An Epidemiologic and Clinical Evaluation of Guillain-Barré Syndrome Reported in Association with the Administration of Swine Influenza Vaccines." *American Journal of Epidemiology* 121, no. 4 (1985): 620–23.

Marks, J. S., and T. J. Halpin. "Guillain-Barré Syndrome in Recipients of A/New Jersey Influenza Vaccine." *Journal of the American Medical Association* 243, no. 24 (1980): 2490–94.

Mickle, Paul. "1976: Fear of a Great Plague." *The Trentonian,* 1998–99.

National Institute of Allergy and Infectious Diseases. "Contact with Pigs Increases Risk of Animal Flu Viruses." www.niaid.nih.gov, Nov. 28, 2005.

Neustadt, R. E., and H. V. Fineburg. "Swine Flu Affair: Decision-Making on a Slippery Disease." Cambridge, Mass.: John F. Kennedy School of Government, 1978.

Retailliau, H. F., A. C. Curtis, G. Storr, G. Caesar, D. L. Eddins, and M.

A. Hattwick. "Illness after Influenza Vaccination Reported through a Nationwide Surveillance System, 1976–1977." *American Journal of Epidemiology* 111, no. 3 (1980): 270–78.

Safranek, T. J., D. N. Lawrence, L. T. Kurland, et al. "Reassessment of the Association between Guillain-Barré Syndrome and Receipt of Swine Influenza Vaccine in 1976–1977: Results of a Two-State Study." *American Journal of Epidemiology* 133, no. 9 (1991): 940–51.

Schonberger, L. B., D. J. Bregman, J. Z. Sullivan-Bolyai, et al. "Guillain-Barré Syndrome Following Vaccination in the National Influenza Immunization Program, United States, 1976–1977." *American Journal of Epidemiology* 110, no. 2 (1979): 105–23.

Schonberger, L. B., E. S. Hurwitz, P. Katona, R. C. Holman, and D. J. Bregman. "Guillain-Barré Syndrome: Its Epidemiology and Associations with Influenza Vaccination." *Annals of Neurology* 9 (Supplement) (1981): 31–38.

Triggle, Nick. "How History Has Taught Us to Fight Flu." BBC News, Oct. 21, 2005.

U.S. Department of Health and Human Services. "Commonly Asked Questions about the National Vaccine Injury Compensation Program." www.HRSA.gov (last updated Dec. 18, 2002).

Chapter 4. A Bird's-Eye View

United Nations Integrated Regional Information Networks, Asia service. "Is Travel to Asia Safe?" www.irinnews.org/Rss/Asia.xml.

Weidensaul, Scott. "Cull of the Wild." *New York Times,* Op-ed, Nov. 30, 2005.

Interviews

Blaker, Ken. President, Experience Asia Tours, Ambassador Worldwide Services. Dec. 3, 2005.

De Haven, Ron, D.V.M. Chief administrator for animal and plant health at the U.S. Dept. of Agriculture. Dec. 2005.

Krushinskie, Elizabeth, D.V.M., Ph.D. Vice president of food safety and production programs at the U.S. Poultry and Egg Association. Dec. 2005.

Swayne, David, D.V.M., Ph.D. Director of the Southeast Poultry Research Lab division of the USDA. Dec. 2005.

Chapter 5. Tamiflu and the Bird Flu Vaccine

Bone, James. "Child Deaths Raise Bird Flu Drug Fears." www.timesonline.co.uk (accessed Nov. 18, 2005).

BIBLIOGRAPHY

Bright, Rick, Marie-jo Medina, Xiyan Xu, Gilda Perez-Oronoz, Teresa R.Wallis, Xiaohong M. Davis, Laura Povinelli, Nancy J. Cox, and Alexander I. Klimov. "Incidence of Adamantane Resistance among Influenza A (H3N2) Viruses Isolated Worldwide from 1994 to 2005: A Cause for Concern." *The Lancet* 366 (2005): 1175–81, DOI:10.1016/S0140-6736(05)67338-2.

Centers for Disease Control and Prevention. "CDC Reports on Antiviral Influenza Drugs." www.cdc.gov (accessed Dec. 5, 2005).

Fauber, John, and Susanne Rust."Bird Flu: Are We Prepared?; The Flu Wars; Race for Vaccine, Anti-Virals Is Lagging." *Milwaukee Journal Sentinel,* Nov. 13, 2005.

Gani, Raymond, Helen Hughes, Douglas Fleming, Thomas Griffin, Jolyon Medlock, and Steve Leach. "Antiviral Drug Use during Influenza Pandemic." Health Protection Agency, Salisbury, Wiltshire, United Kingdom; and Royal College of General Practitioners, Harborne, Birmingham, United Kingdom. www.cdc.gov/ncidod/EID/vol11no09/pdfs/04-1344.pdf.

Macpherson, Kitta. "Vaccine Researchers Hope to Benefit from Bush Flu Plan." Newhouse News Service, Nov. 3, 2005.

Minneapolis Star Tribune. "Federal Health Officials Say Tamiflu Is Safe." Nov. 18, 2005.

National Institute of Allergy and Infectious Diseases and the National Institutes of Health. "Flu Drugs." http://www.niaid.nih.gov/factsheets/fludrugs.htm.

Pellerin, Cheryl. "Bird Flu Needs Better, Modern Vaccine Production Methods." usinfo.state.gov/gi/Archive/2005/Oct/21-397391.html.

Physicians Desk Reference 2005. "Tamiflu."

Plotkin, S. L., and S. A. Plotkin. "A Short History of Vaccination," *Vaccines,* 4th ed. Philadelphia: W. B. Saunders Co., 2002.

Siegel, Marc. "Desperate for Cipro." *New York Times,* Oct. 21, 2001.

Yen, Hui-Ling, Arnold S. Monto, Robert G. Webster, and Elena A. Govorkova. "Tamiflu Helps Mice Survive H5N1." St. Jude's Children's Research Hospital in Memphis, *Zoonotic Disease,* CIDRAP, July 18, 2005.

CHAPTER 6. OUR CULTURE OF FEAR

Allan, Stuart. *Media, Risk, and Science.* Berkshire, UK: Open University Press, 2002.

American Psychiatric Association. *Diagnostic and Statistical Manual of Mental Disorders.* Arlington: American Psychiatric Association, 1994.

Barad, Mark, Chris Cain, and Ashley Blouin. "L-type Voltage Gated Calcium Channels Are Required for Extinction of Fear." *Journal of Neuroscience* 22, no. 20 (Oct. 15, 2002): 9113–21.

Barber, Benjamin. *Fear's Empire: War, Terrorism, and Democracy.* New York: W. W. Norton, 2003.

Barsky, Ahern. "Therapy for Hypochondriasis: A Randomized Controlled Trial." *Journal of the American Medical Association* 291, no. 12 (2004): 1464.

Bobbitt, Philip. "Being Clear about Present Dangers." *New York Times,* Aug. 11, 2004.

Bradley, Walter. *Neurology in Clinical Practice.* Burlington, Vt.: Butterworth-Heinemann, 1996.

Braunwald, Eugene, et al. *Harrison's Principles of Internal Medicine,* 15th ed. New York: McGraw-Hill, 2001.

Bremner, J. D. *Does Stress Damage the Brain? Understanding Trauma-Related Disorders from a Neurological Perspective.* New York: W. W. Norton & Co., 2002.

Brooks, Renana. "A Nation of Victims." *The Nation,* June 30, 2003.

Bumiller, Elisabeth. "Bush Makes Danger His Campaign Theme." *New York Times,* Jan. 25, 2004.

Bush, George W. Interview by Tim Russert, *Meet the Press,* NBC, Feb. 7, 2004, aired Feb. 8, 2004. NBC News transcript.

Cohl, H. Aaron. *Are We Scaring Ourselves to Death? How Pessimism, Paranoia, and a Misguided Media Are Leading Us toward Disaster.* New York: St. Martin's Press, 1997.

Cooper, Joel. "What's Inside the Voter's Mind?" *Newsday,* Oct. 31, 2004.

Corey, Robin. *Fear: The History of a Political Idea.* New York: Oxford University Press, 2004.

De Becker, Gavin. *Fear Less: Real Truth about Risk, Safety, and Security in a Time of Terrorism.* New York: Little Brown, 2002.

———. *The Gift of Fear.* New York: Little Brown, 1997.

Descartes, René. *The Passions of the Soul: An English Translation of Les Passions De L'Ame* (1649). Trans. Stephen Voss. Indianapolis: Hackett Publishing Company, 1990.

Diehl, Jackson. "Dubious Threat, Expensive Defense." *Washington Post,* Apr. 26, 2004.

Duenwald, Mary. "A New Era in Treating Imaginary Ills." *New York Times,* Mar. 30, 2004.

Easterbrook, Gregg. "In an Age of Terror, Safety Is Relative." *New York Times,* June 27, 2004.

———. "The Smart Way to Be Scared." *New York Times,* Feb. 16, 2003.

Ekman, Paul. *Emotions Revealed: Recognizing Faces and Feelings to Improve Communication and Emotional Life.* New York: Times Books, 2003.

Fowles, Jinnet B., Allan C. Kind, et al. "Patients' Interest in Reading Their Medical Record, Relation with Clinical and Sociodemographic

Characteristics and Patients' Approach to Health Care." *Archives of Internal Medicine* 164 (Apr. 12, 2004): 793–800.

Fox, James Alan, and Jack Levin. "Media Exaggerate Sniper Threat." *USA Today,* Dec. 9, 2003.

Furedi, Frank. *Culture of Fear: Risk-Taking and the Morality of Low Expectations.* New York: Continuum, 2002.

Garcia, Rene, Richard Thompson, Michel Baudry, and Rose Marie Vouimba. "The Amygdala Modulates Prefrontal Cortex Activity Relative to Conditioned Fear." *Nature* 402 (Nov. 18, 1999): 294–6.

Glassner, Barry. *The Culture of Fear: Why Americans Are Afraid of All the Wrong Things.* New York: Basic Books, 1999.

Greenberg, Jeff, Andy Martens, Eva Jonas, Donna Eisenstadt, Thomas Pyszczynski, and Sheldon Solomon. "Psychological Defense in Anticipation of Anxiety: Eliminating the Potential for Anxiety Eliminates the Effect of Mortality Salience on Worldview Defense." *Psychological Science* vol.14, issue 5 (Sept. 2003): 516.

Groopman, Jerome. *The Anatomy of Hope: How People Prevail in the Face of Illness.* New York: Random House, 2003.

Harwood, John. "Theme of Fear Plays Key Role in Election and May Favor Bush." *Wall Street Journal,* Sept. 1, 2004.

Hind, Rick, and David Halperin. "Lots of Chemicals, Little Reaction." *New York Times,* Sept. 22, 2004.

Honig, Robin Marantz. "The Quest to Forget." *New York Times Magazine,* Apr. 4, 2004.

Ignatieff, Michael. *The Lesser Evil: Political Ethics in an Age of Terror.* Princeton: Princeton University Press, 2004.

Jeffers, Susan. *Feel the Fear and Do It Anyway.* New York: Harcourt, 1987.

———. *Feel the Fear . . . and Beyond: Master the Techniques for Doing It Anyway.* New York: Ballantine Books, 1998.

Kass, Leon. *Beyond Therapy: Biotechnology and the Pursuit of Happiness.* New York: Regan Books, 2003.

Kipnis, Jonathon, Hagit Cohen, Michal Cordan, et al. "T Cell Deficiency Leads to Cognitive Dysfunction, Implications for Therapeutic Vaccination for Schizophrenia and Other Psychiatric Conditions." *Proceedings of the National Academy of Sciences,* May 2004.

Krauthammer, Charles. "The Case for Fearmongering." *Time,* Oct. 18, 2004.

Krugman, Paul. "To Tell the Truth." *New York Times,* May 28, 2004.

Landau, Mark J., Sheldon Solomon, and Jeff Greenberg. "Deliver Us from Evil: The Effects of Mortality Salience and Reminders of 9/11 on Support for President George W. Bush." *Personality and Social Psychology Bulletin* 30, no. 9 (2004): 1136–50.

Landro, Laura. "Disaster Medicine Becomes a Specialty." *Wall Street Journal,* Aug. 12, 2004.

LeDoux, Joseph. *The Emotional Brain: The Mysterious Underpinnings of Emotional Life.* New York: Simon and Schuster, 1996.

Longeman, Jere. *Among the Heroes: United Flight 93 and the Passengers and Crew Who Fought Back.* New York: HarperCollins, 2002.

Low, Phillip. *Clinical Autonomic Disorders.* Philadelphia: Lippincott Williams & Wilkins, 1997.

Manning, Anita. "Smallpox Vaccination Plan Ceased." *USA Today,* Oct. 15, 2003.

McCarty, Richard, Greti Aguilera, Esther L. Sabban, and Richard Kvetnansky, eds. *Stress: Neural, Endocrine, and Molecular Studies.* Taylor & Francis, Sept. 2001.

Meagher, Mary W., Randolph C. Arnau, and Jamie L. Rudy. "Pain and Emotion: Effects of Affective Picture Modulation." *Psychosomatic Medicine* 63 (2001): 79–90.

Milad, M. R., and G. J. Quirk. "Neurons in Medial Prefrontal Cortex Signal Memory for Fear Extinction." *Nature* 240 (Nov. 7, 2002): 70–74.

Mitchell, Luke. "A Run on Terror." *Harper's Magazine,* Mar. 2004.

Morgan, M. Granger, Baruch Fischhoff, Ann Bostrom, and Cynthia J. Atman. *Risk Communication: A Mental Models Approach.* New York: Cambridge University Press, 2002.

New York Times. "The Face of Scare Politics" (editorial). Dec. 11, 2003.

Nuland, Sherwin. *How We Die: Reflections on Life's Final Chapter.* New York: Knopf, 1994.

Nunberg, Geoffrey. "The -Ism Schism: How Much Wallop Can a Simple Word Pack?" *New York Times,* July 11, 2004.

Olsson, Andreas, and Elizabeth A. Phelps. "Learned Fear of 'Unseen' Faces after Pavlovian, Observational, and Instructed Fear," *Psychological Science* 15, no. 12 (Dec. 2004): 822–28(7).

Pan, Michael, Amanda Terkel, Robert Boorstin, P. J. Crowley, and Nigel Holmes. "Op-Chart: Safety Second." *New York Times,* Aug. 8, 2004.

Peters, Ralph. "Not So Innocent, Media's Devastating Impact." *New York Post,* Oct. 8, 2003.

Phelps, Elizabeth. "Extinction Learning in Humans: Role of the Amygdala and vmPFC." *Neuron* 43 (Sept. 16, 2004): 897–905.

Purnick, Joyce. "Rationing Fear and Assessing Vulnerability." *New York Times,* Aug. 2, 2004.

Pyszczynski, Thomas A., Sheldon Solomon, and Jeff Greenberg. *In the Wake of 9/11: The Psychology of Terror.* Washington, D.C.: American Psychological Association, 2002.

Rich, Frank. "The Best Goebbels of All?" *New York Times,* June 27, 2004.

Robin, Corey. "When Fear Is a Joint Venture." *Washington Post,* Oct. 24, 2004.

Ropeik, David, and George Gray. *Risk: A Practical Guide for Deciding What's Really Safe and What's Really Dangerous in the World around You.* New York: Houghton Mifflin, 2002.

Ropeik, David, and Nigel Holmes. "Never Bitten, Twice Shy: The Real Dangers of Summer." *New York Times,* Aug. 9, 2003.

Rothstein, Edward. "Is Fear Itself the Enemy? Or Perhaps the Lack of It?" *New York Times,* Feb. 14, 2004.

Sabban, Esther L., and Kvetnansky, Richard. "Stress-Triggered Activation of Gene Expression in Catecholaminergic Systems: Dynamics of Transcriptional Events." *Trends in Neurosciences* 24, no. 2 (Feb. 2001).

Sapadin, Linda. *Master Your Fears: How to Triumph Over Your Worries and Get On with Your Life.* Hoboken: John Wiley & Sons, 2004.

Sapolsky, Robert M. "Glucocorticoids and Hippocampal Atrophy in Neuropsychiatric Disorders." *Archives of General Psychiatry* 57, no. 10 (2000): 925–35.

———. *A Primate's Memoir: A Neuroscientist's Unconventional Life among the Baboons.* New York: Scribner, 2001.

Schneier, Bruce. *Beyond Fear.* New York: Copernicus, 2003.

Shumyatsky, G. P., G. Malleret, S. Vronskaya, M. Hatton, L. Hampton, J. F. Battey, C. Dulac, E. R. Kandel, and V. Y. Bolshakov. "Identification of a Signaling Network in Lateral Nucleus of Amygdala Important for Inhibiting Memory Specifically Related to Learned Fear." *Cell* 111, no. 6 (Dec. 13, 2002): 905–18.

Siegel, Marc. "Diary of a 9/11 Doctor." *Diversion* (Doctors Who Volunteer), Apr. 15, 2002.

———. "Fear Created by the Unknown." *Los Angeles Times* Health section, Jan. 26, 2004.

———. "He Found His Own Path Back to Good Health." *Los Angeles Times* Health section, June 28, 2004.

———. "How Terror Fears Make You Sick." *USA Today,* Oct. 14, 2004.

———. "I'm Sorry, Your Illness Is Coded for Only 15 Minutes." *Washington Post,* Sept. 14, 2003.

———. "Terrorism Is Everywhere. Only It Isn't." *USA Today,* Op-ed, Aug. 9, 2005.

———. "When Doctors Say Don't and the Patient Says Do." *New York Times,* Oct. 29, 2002.

Slater, Lauren. "The Cruelest Cure." *New York Times Magazine,* Nov. 2, 2003.

Slovic, Paul. *The Perception of Risk.* London: Earthscan, 2000.

Solomon, Sheldon, Jeff Greenberg, and Tom Pyszczynski. "Reminders of Death Increase the Need for Psychological Security and Therefore the Appeal of Leaders Who Emphasize the Greatness of the Nation and a Heroic Victory over Evil." *Psychological Science* 15, no. 12 (Dec. 2004).

Sunstein, Cass, *Risk and Reason: Safety, Law, and the Environment.* New York: Cambridge University Press, 2002.

Tulloch, John, and Deborah Lupton. *Risk and Everyday Life.* Thousand Oaks, Calif.: Sage Publications, 2003.

Whelan, Elizabeth M. *Toxic Terror: The Truth behind the Cancer Scares.* Amherst, N.Y.: Prometheus Books, 1993.

Wright, Scott M., David E. Kern, Ken Kolodner, Donna M. Howard, and Frederick L. Brancati. "Attributes of Excellent Attending-Physician Role Models," *New England Journal of Medicine* 339, no. 27 (Dec. 31, 1998): 1986–93.

INTERVIEWS

Jolly, Chris, Ph.D. Professor of anthropology, New York University, telephone interview, Dec. 18, 2003.

LeDoux, Joseph, Ph.D. Professor of neuroscience, New York University, phone interview, Dec. 17, 2003.

Mann, John, M.D. Director of neuroscience at the New York State Psychiatric Institute, telephone interview, Jan. 22, 2004.

Phelps, Elizabeth, Ph.D. Associate professor of psychology and neuroscience, New York University, e-mail correspondence, Dec. 2004; telephone interview, Dec. 30, 2004.

Sabban, Esther, Ph.D. Professor and graduate program director, Department of Biochemistry and Molecular Biology, New York Medical College, phone interview, Dec. 22, 2003.

Yehuda, Rachel, Ph.D. Professor of psychiatry at Mt. Sinai School of Medicine, phone interview, Dec. 29, 2003.

CHAPTER 7. SARS

Altman, Lawrence K. "New SARS Reports, New Questions on Tracking." *New York Times,* Jan. 2, 2004.

———. "Step by Step, Scientists Track Mystery Ailment." *New York Times,* Apr. 1, 2003.

———. "What Is the Next Plague?" *New York Times,* Nov. 11, 2003.

Associated Press. "CDC: SARS Fears Could Swamp Emergency Rooms This Winter." Oct. 2003.

BBC. "China Guards Against SARS." Oct. 13, 2003.

Bradsher, Keith. "From Tourism to High Finance, Mysterious Illness Spreads Havoc." *New York Times,* Apr. 2, 2003.

———. "Illness Takes a Toll on Hotels in Asia." *New York Times,* Apr. 4, 2003.

Callan, Sara. "Sorry, Fear of Illness Isn't Covered—Travel Insurance Can Help If You're Too Sick to Go, Not If You're Too Scared." *Wall Street Journal*, Apr. 3, 2003.

Centers for Disease Control and Prevention. "Preliminary Clinical Description of Severe Acute Respiratory Syndrome" (health update). Mar. 22, 2003.

Chase, Marilyn. "Epidemics Take Variety of Courses, History Offers Some Clues to How the SARS Outbreak May Grow—or Dissipate." *Wall Street Journal*, Apr. 4, 2003.

Gerberding, Julie Louise. "Faster . . . But Fast Enough? Responding to the Epidemic of Severe Acute Respiratory Syndrome." *New England Journal of Medicine*, Apr. 2, 2003.

Grady, Denise. "Fear Reigns as Dangerous Mystery Illness Spreads in Asia and Beyond." *New York Times*, Apr. 7, 2003.

———. "SARS Is New and It Kills, but How Dangerous Is It?" *New York Times*, Apr. 6, 2003.

Harmon, Amy. "Public Confronts New Virus on Laymen's Terms." *New York Times*, Apr. 6, 2003.

Lieber, Ron, and Scott Neuman. "Airlines Step Up Effort to Prevent SARS." *Wall Street Journal*, Apr. 3, 2003.

McNeil, Donald G. Jr., and Lawrence K. Altman. "China Admits to Having More of Mystery Illness." *New York Times*, Apr. 3, 2003.

New York Times. "Preparing for SARS [Return]" (editorial). Oct. 26, 2003.

Normile, D. "Second Lab Accident Fuels Fears about SARS." *Science* 303 (2004): 26.

Parker-Pope, Tara. "Reality Check: Asian Mystery Disease Is Scary Mostly Because It's New." *Wall Street Journal*, Apr. 2, 2003.

Pottinger, Matt, Betsy McKay, and Elena Cherney. "Treating a Medical Mystery." *Wall Street Journal*, Apr. 3, 2003.

Siegel, Marc. "Hysteria Spreads Faster than SARS." *Boston Globe*, Apr. 5, 2003.

———. "A Virus of Fear." *New York Times*, May 4, 2003.

Svoboda, Tomislav, et al. "Public Health Measures to Control the Spread of the Severe Acute Respiratory Syndrome during the Outbreak in Toronto." *New England Journal of Medicine* 350, no. 3 (June 3, 2004): 2352–61.

Wall Street Journal. "Divergent Asian Responses Show Difficulties in Dealing With SARS." Apr. 7, 2003.

———. "Health Experts Go to the Source of SARS Virus—Team Is in Southern China As Cases Multiply in Asia; Toronto Extends Quarantine." Apr. 4, 2003.

Weinstein, Robert A. "Planning for Epidemics—The Lessons of SARS."

New England Journal of Medicine 350, no. 3 (June 3, 2004): 2332–4.

Wonacott, Peter, Betsy McKay, David P. Hamilton. "Fear of SARS Rises as Cases—and Rumors—Spread." *Wall Street Journal,* Apr. 2, 2003.

Wong, Edward. "Stop-and-Go Traffic on a Global Scale." *New York Times,* Apr. 6, 2003.

CHAPTER 8. THE OTHER FLU

Altman, Lawrence K. "Despite Lacking Latest Virus, Flu Vaccine Is Thought to Work." *New York Times,* Nov. 18, 2003.

Associated Press. "Beating the Flu: A Spray or a Shot?" Sept. 23, 2003.

——— "Hospitals Restrict Visitors to Prevent Infection." Dec. 12, 2003.

BBC. "Cure for Killer Flu Discovered." Oct. 20, 2003.

Centers for Disease Control and Prevention. "Prevention and Control of Influenza: Recommendations of the Advisory Committee on Immunization Practices." *Morbidity and Mortality Weekly Report,* no. RR-4 (1999): 48.

———. Weekly Influenza Activity Estimates," week ending Nov. 29, 2003. www.cdc.gov/flu/weekly/usmap.htm.

———. "What Everyone Should Know about Flu and the Flu Vaccine" (fact sheet). www.cdc.gov (accessed Oct. 6, 2004).

Clover, R. D., T. Abell, L. A. Becker, et al. "Family Functioning and Stress as Predictors of Influenza B Infection." *Journal of Family Practice* 28 (1989): 535–39.

Cox, N. J., and K. Subbarao. "Influenza." *Lancet* 354 (1999): 1277–82.

Kenworthy, Tom. "Even Though Flu Season 'Is Going Gangbusters,' It Could End Quickly Too." *USA Today,* Dec. 10, 2003.

Lui, K.-J., and A. P. Kendal. "Impact of Influenza Epidemics on Mortality in the United States from October 1972 to May 1985." *American Journal of Public Health* 77 (1987): 712–16.

Manning, Anita. "Universal Flu Shots Considered." *USA Today,* Feb. 24, 2004.

National Institutes of Health, Office of Communications and Public Liaison, National Instutute of Allergy and Infections Diseases. "Flu Drugs." www.niaid.nih.gov/factsheets/flu.htm (accessed June 17, 2003).

Pauling, Linus. *Vitamin C, the Common Cold, and the Flu.* San Francisco: W. H. Freeman & Company, 1976.

Pearson, Helen. "Diluted Flu Vaccine Works Well." *Nature Online,* www.nature.com/news/2004/041101/pf/041101-13_pf.html (accessed Nov. 4. 2004).

Schmid, M. L., G. Kudesia, S. Wake, and R. C. Read. "Prospective Comparative Study of Culture Specimens and Methods in Diagnosing Influenza in Adults." *British Medical Journal* 316 (1998): 275.

Siegel, Marc. "Ho-hum Killer Creates Real Risk." *USA Today,* Oct. 16, 2003.

Simonsen, L., L. B. Schonberger, D. F. Stroup, N. H. Arden, and N. J. Cox. "The Impact of Influenza on Mortality in the USA," in *Options for the Control of Influenza III*, ed. L. E. Brown, A. W. Hampson, and R. G. Webster. Amsterdam: Elsevier Publishing Co., 1996: 26–33.

Tuller, David. "Promoting Flu Shots for All." *New York Times,* Oct. 14, 2003.

Winquist, Andrea G., Keija Fukuda, Carolyn B. Bridges, and Nancy J. Cox. "Neuraminidase Inhibitors for Treatment of Influenza A and B Infections." Centers for Disease Control, Division of Viral and Rickettsial Diseases, National Center for Infectious Disease. Dec. 17, 1999 / 48(RR14): 1–9.

World Health Organization. Communicable Disease Surveillance and Response, WHO Global Influenza Surveillance Network. www.who.int/csr/disease/influenza/ (accessed Oct. 6, 2004).

———. Flunet activity map showing "hot areas" in Chile and Australia 8/24/03–9/27/03. www.phac-aspc.gc.ca/fluwatch/03-04/w36_03.

Yale New Haven Health. "Complementary Medicine: Information about Complementary and Alternative Medical Therapies to Influenza." www.yalenewhavenhealth.org/library/healthguide/en-us/Cam/topic.asp?hwid=hn-1398005 (accessed Jan. 15, 2004).

Zambon, M. "Laboratory Diagnosis of Influenza," in *Textbook of Influenza*, ed. K. G. Nicholson, R. G. Webster, and A. J. Hay. Oxford: Blackwell Science, 1998: 291–313.

CHAPTER 9. DO WE KNOW A PANDEMIC WHEN WE SEE ONE?
AIDS VERSUS BIRD FLU

Agence France-Presse. "Beijing Criticized for Slow Progress in War on AIDS." Nov. 22, 2005.

Altman, Lawrence K. "As Bird Flu Spreads, Global Health Weaknesses Are Exposed." *New York Times,* Feb. 3, 2004.

———. "Avian Flu Said to Be Resistant to a Main Flu-Fighting Drug." *New York Times,* Jan. 25, 2004.

———. "Experts Urge Bird Vaccination Against Flu." *New York Times,* Feb. 6, 2004.

———. "U.S. Issues Its First Plan for Responding to a Flu Pandemic." *New York Times,* Aug. 26, 2004.

American Lung Association. "Flu." www.lungusa.org (accessed Oct. 23, 2004).

Associated Press. "Bird Flu Surfaces in Delaware." Feb. 6, 2004.

Barry, John. "History Offers Lessons on Flu's Threats." *USA Today,* Feb. 10, 2004.

BIBLIOGRAPHY

BBC. "1918 Killer Flu Secrets Revealed." Feb. 5, 2004.

Bradsher, Keith, and Lawrence K.Altman. "Thais Infected with Bird Flu; Virus Spreads." *New York Times,* Jan. 24, 2004.

Broder, John. "At Entry Points, on the Lookout for Symptoms." *New York Times,* Nov. 22, 2005.

Brown, David. "This Year's Potential Pandemic, HHS Calls for Plan to Counter Threat of Flu." *Washington Post,* Aug. 25, 2004.

Bundy, Jennifer. "Thousands Line Up for Desperate Shot at Flu Vaccine." Associated Press, Oct. 16, 2004.

Centers for Disease Control and Prevention. "Information on Influenza Anti-Viral Drugs." *Morbidity and Mortality Weekly Report,* www.cdc.gov/mmwr (accessed Oct. 31, 2004).

Crispin, Shawn, Margot Cohen, and Timothy Mapes. "Bird-Flu Outbreak Revives Concerns Stirred by SARS." *Wall Street Journal,* Jan. 28, 2004.

Davis, Matthew. "The Failure to Deal with the Flu." *Los Angeles Times,* October 8, 2004.

Etter, Lauren, "Hot Topic: Avian Flu: Pandemic on the Horizon?" *Weekend Wall Street Journal,* Oct. 22–23, 2005.

Grady, Denise. "Before Shortage of Flu Vaccine, Many Warnings." *New York Times,* Oct. 17, 2004.

Haney, Daniel Q. "Experts: Bird Flu Could Become Epidemic." Associated Press, Jan. 24, 2004.

Harris, Gardiner, "U.S. Bans Imports of Some Canadian Poultry," *New York Times,* Nov. 22, 2005.

Heikkinen, Terho, Aimo Salmi, and Olli Ruuskanen. "Comparative Study of Nasopharyngeal Aspirate and Nasal Swab Ppecimens for Detection of Influenza." *British Medical Journal* 322, no. 7279 (Jan. 20, 2001): 138.

Kolata, Gina, "Experts Unlock Clues to Spread of 1918 Flu Virus." *New York Times,* A1, Oct. 6, 2005.

Maier, Thomas. "Flu Vaccine: Two Pictures of Health." *Newsday,* Oct. 24, 2004.

Manning, Anita. "Demand for Flu Shots Takes Off." *USA Today,* Oct. 8, 2004.

Matsumoto, K. "Anti-influenza Drugs and the Standard of Use." *Nippon Rinsho* 58, no. 11 (Nov. 2000): 2283–97.

McFadden, Robert D. "Frustration and Fear Reign Over Flu Shots." *New York Times,* Oct. 16, 2004.

New York Times. "An Influenza Vaccine Debacle" (editorial). Oct. 20, 2004.

———. "The Perplexing Pandemic Flu Plan" (editorial). Nov. 20, 2005.

———. "Preparing for the Bird Flu." (editorial). Dec. 17, 2003.

———. "The Spread of Avian Influenza" (editorial). Jan. 30, 2004.

Parker-Pope, Tara. "Do You Really Need to Get a Flu Shot?" *Wall Street Journal,* Oct. 26, 2004.

Regaldo, Antonio. "Scientists Rush to Create Vaccine for Bird Flu—Just in Case." *Wall Street Journal,* Jan. 28, 2004.

Ricks, Delthia. "Flu Vaccine Promising." *Newsday,* Oct. 12, 2006.

———. "Bracing for a Worst-Case Scenario, Health Officials Will Outline a Preparedness Plan if Deadly Avian Flu Strain Goes Global, and to U.S." *Newsday,* Nov. 2, 2005.

Ross, Emma. "WHO: Unsafe Handling Raises Bird Flu Risk." Associated Press, Mar. 3, 2004.

Siegel, Marc. "Flu Tips." *Family Circle,* Nov. 30, 2004.

———. Letter to the editor on Gina Kolata's Oct. 6th article. *New York Times,* Oct. 13, 2005.

———. "A Tough Choice: Who Gets the Shot." *Los Angeles Times,* Oct. 25, 2004.

———. "Vaccine Poker." *The Nation,* Oct. 14, 2004.

Wall Street Journal. "The Needless Worry over Influenza Vaccine." Sept. 14, 2004.

World Health Organization. "Epidemic and Pandemic Alert and Response (EPR)." www.who.int.

Wysocki, Bernard Jr. "U.S. Sees Need to Better Prepare Against Avian Flu." *Wall Street Journal,* Oct. 6, 2005.

Wysocki, Bernard Jr., and Betsy Mckay. "Flu-Vaccine Shortage Signals U.S. Vulnerability to Pandemic." *Wall Street Journal,* Oct. 8, 2004.

CHAPTER 10. PERSPECTIVES

Reuters. "Worst-Case Flu Scenario." Dec. 6, 2005.

Siegel, Marc. "Afraid of the Bird Flu? The Worse Virus Is Fear: Why a Pandemic That Isn't Even Here Is Driving My Patients Crazy." Brainstorm, *Fortune,* Nov. 28, 2005.

———. "Alive and Well: The Fear Epidemic." *USA Today,* Op-ed, Oct. 17, 2005.

———. "Can We Cure Fear?" *Scientific American Mind,* Dec. 2005.

———. "Don't Worry, Be Healthy: Fear Is More Likely to Get You Than the Avian Flu." *Slate,* Sept. 13, 2005.

———. "An Epidemic of Overreaction" *Los Angeles Times,* Op-ed, Oct. 11, 2005.

———. "Flighty Flu Fears." *New York Post,* Op-ed, Oct. 12, 2005.

———. "Flu Fear for the Birds." *New York Post,* Op-ed, Aug. 15, 2005.

———. Interview by Esther Pan. Council on Foreign Relations, Aug. 17, 2005.

———. "The Irony of Fear: Irrational Health Anxieties Boost Your Risk of the Conditions You Should Fear the Most." *Washington Post*, Aug. 30, 2005, HE01.

Weeks, Linton. "Fear Factory." *Washington Post*, Style section, Dec. 5, 2005.